Headaches

Mary Kittredge

Introduction by C. Everett Koop, M.D., Sc.D.
Former Surgeon General, U.S. Public Health Service

Foreword by Sandra Thurman
Director, Office of National AIDS Policy, The White House

CHELSEA HOUSE PUBLISHERS
Philadelphia

The goal of 21ST CENTURY HEALTH AND WELLNESS is to provide general information in the ever-changing areas of physiology, psychology, and related medical issues. The titles in this series are not intended to take the place of the professional advice of a physician or other health-care professional.

Chelsea House Publishers
EDITOR IN CHIEF: Stephen Reginald
PRODUCTION MANAGER: Pamela Loos
ART DIRECTOR: Sara Davis
DIRECTOR OF PHOTOGRAPHY: Judy Hasday
MANAGING EDITOR: James D. Gallagher
SENIOR PRODUCTION EDITOR: J. Christopher Higgins
ASSISTANT EDITOR: Anne Hill
PRODUCTION SERVICES: Pre-Press Company, Inc.
COVER DESIGNER/ILLUSTRATOR: Emiliano Begnardi

The Chelsea House World Wide Web site address is http://www.chelseahouse.com

1 3 5 7 9 8 6 4 2

Library of Congress Cataloging-in-Publication Data

Kittredge, Mary, 1949–
Headaches / Mary Kittredge ; introduction by C. Everett Koop ; foreword by Sandra Thurman.
p. cm. — (21st century health and wellness)
Includes bibliographical references and index.
Summary: Discusses headaches—causes, treatments, and various kinds.
ISBN 0-7910-5981-2
1. Headache—Juvenile literature. [1. Headache] I. Title. II. Series.

RB128.K57 2001
616.8'491—dc21   00-027516

CONTENTS

- AIDS
- Allergies
- The Circulatory System
- The Common Cold
- Death & Dying
- The Digestive System
- The Endocrine System
- Headaches
- Holistic Medicine
- The Human Body: An Overview
- The Immune System
- Mononucleosis and Other Infectious Diseases
- Organ Transplants
- Pregnancy & Birth
- The Respiratory System
- Sexually Transmitted Diseases
- Skin Disorders
- Sports Medicine
- Stress Management

PREVENTION AND EDUCATION: THE KEYS TO GOOD HEALTH

C. Everett Koop, M.D., Sc.D.
FORMER SURGEON GENERAL,
U.S. Public Health Service

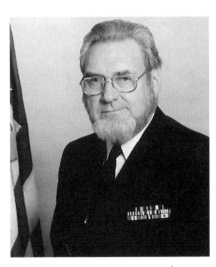

The issue of health education has received particular attention in recent years because of the presence of AIDS in the news. But our response to this particular tragedy points up a number of broader issues that doctors, public health officials, educators, and the public face. In particular, it spotlights the importance of sound health education for citizens of all ages.

Over the past 35 years, this country has been able to achieve dramatic declines in the death rates from heart disease, stroke, accidents, and—for people under the age of 45—cancer. Today, Americans generally eat better and take better care of themselves than ever before. Thus, with the help of modern science and technology, they have a better chance of surviving serious—even catastrophic—illnesses. In 1996, the life expectancy of Americans reached an all-time high of 76.1 years. That's the good news.

The flip side of this advance has special significance for young adults. According to a report issued in 1998 by the U.S. Department of Health and Human Services, levels of wealth and education in the United States are directly correlated with our population's health. The more money Americans make and the more years of schooling they have, the better their health will be. Furthermore, income inequality increased in the U.S. between 1970 and 1996. Basically, the rich got richer—people in high income brackets had greater increases in the amount of money made than did those at low income levels. In addition, the report indicated that children under 18 are more likely to live in poverty than the population as a whole.

Family income rises with each higher level of education for both men and women from every ethnic and racial background. Life expectancy, too, is related to family income. People with lower incomes tend to die at younger ages than people from more affluent homes. What all this means is that health is a factor of wealth and education, both of which need to be improved for all Americans if the promise of life, liberty, and the pursuit of happiness is to include an equal chance for good health.

The health of young people is further threatened by violent death and injury, alcohol and drug abuse, unwanted pregnancies, and sexually transmitted diseases. Adolescents are particularly vulnerable because they are beginning to explore their own sexuality and perhaps to experiment with drugs and alcohol. We need to educate young people to avoid serious dangers to their health. The price of neglect is high.

Even for the population as a whole, health is still far from what it could be. Why? Most death and disease are attributed to four broad elements: inadequacies in the health-care system, behavioral factors or unhealthy lifestyles, environmental hazards, and human biological factors. These categories are also influenced by individual resources. For example, low birth weight and infant mortality are more common among the children of less educated mothers. Likewise, women with more education are more likely to obtain prenatal care during pregnancy. Mothers with fewer than 12 years of education are almost 10 times more likely to smoke during pregnancy—and new studies find excessive aggression later in life as well as other physical ailments among the children of smokers. In short, poor people with less education are more likely to smoke cigarettes, which endangers health and shortens the life span. About a third of the children who begin smoking will eventually have their lives cut short because of this practice.

Similarly, poor children are exposed more often to environmental lead, which causes a wide range of physical and mental problems. Sedentary lifestyles are also more common among teens with lower family income than among wealthier adolescents. Being overweight—a condition associated with physical inactivity as well as excessive caloric intake—is also more common among poor, non-Hispanic, white adolescents. Children from rich families are more likely to have health insurance. Therefore, they are more apt to receive vaccinations and other forms of early preventative medicine and treatment. The bottom line is that kids from lower income groups receive less adequate health care.

To be sure, some diseases are still beyond the control of even the most advanced medical techniques that our richest citizens can afford. Despite yearnings that are as old as the human race itself, there is no "fountain of youth" to prevent aging and death. Still, solutions are available for many of the problems that undermine sound health. In a word, that solution is prevention. Prevention, which includes health promotion and education, can save lives, improve the quality of life, and, in the long run, save money.

In the United States, organized public health activities and preventative medicine have a long history. Important milestones include the improvement of sanitary procedures and the development of pasteurized milk in the late-19th century, and the introduction in the mid-20th century of effective vaccines against polio, measles, German measles, mumps, and other once-rampant diseases. Internationally, organized public health efforts began on a wide-scale basis with the International Sanitary Conference of 1851, to which 12 nations sent representatives. The World Health Organization, founded in 1948, continues these efforts under the aegis of the United Nations, with particular emphasis on combating communicable diseases and the training of health-care workers.

Despite these accomplishments, much remains to be done in the field of prevention. For too long, we have had a medical system that is science and technology-based, and focuses essentially on illness and mortality. It is now patently obvious that both the social and the economic costs of such a system are becoming insupportable.

Implementing prevention and its corollaries, health education and health promotion, is the job of several groups of people. First, the medical and scientific professions need to continue basic scientific research, and here we are making considerable progress. But increased concern with prevention will also have a decided impact on how primary-care doctors practice medicine. With a shift to health-based rather than morbidity-based medicine, the role of the "new physician" includes a healthy dose of patient education.

Second, practitioners of the social and behavioral sciences— psychologists, economists, and city planners along with lawyers, business leaders, and government officials—must solve the practical and ethical dilemmas confronting us: poverty, crime, civil rights, literacy, education, employment, housing, sanitation, environmental protection, health-care delivery systems, and so forth. All of these issues affect public health.

Third is the public at large. We consider this group to be important in any movement. Fourth, and the linchpin in this effort, is the public health profession: doctors, epidemiologists, teachers—who must harness the professional expertise of the first two groups and the common sense and cooperation of the third: the public. They must define the problems statistically and qualitatively and then help set priorities for finding solutions.

To a very large extent, improving health statistics is the responsibility of every individual. So let's consider more specifically what the role of the individual should be and why health education is so important. First, and most obviously, individuals can protect themselves from illness and injury and thus minimize the need for professional medical care. They can eat a nutritious diet; get adequate exercise; avoid tobacco, alcohol, and drugs; and take prudent steps to avoid accidents. The proverbial "apple a day keeps the doctor away" is not so far from the truth, after all.

Second, individuals should actively participate in their own medical care. They should schedule regular medical and dental checkups. If an illness or injury develops, they should know when to treat themselves and when to seek professional help. To gain the maximum benefit from any medical treatment, individuals must become partners in treatment. For instance, they should understand the effects and side effects of medications. I counsel young physicians that there is no such thing as too much information when talking with patients. But the corollary is the patient must know enough about the nuts and bolts of the healing process to understand what the doctor is telling him or her. That responsibility is at least partially the patient's.

Education is equally necessary for us to understand the ethical and public policy issues in health care today. Sometimes individuals will encounter these issues in making decisions about their own treatment or that of family members. Other citizens may encounter them as jurors in medical malpractice cases. But we all become involved, indirectly, when we elect our public officials, from school board members to the president. Should surrogate parenting be legal? To what extent is drug testing desirable, legal, or necessary? Should there be public funding for family planning, hospitals, various types of medical research, and medical care for the indigent? How should we allocate scant technological resources, such as kidney dialysis and organ transplants? What is the proper role of government in protecting the rights of patients?

What are the broad goals of public health in the United States today? The Public Health Service has defined these goals in terms of mortality, education, and health improvement. It identified 15 major concerns: controlling high blood pressure, improving family planning, pregnancy care and infant health, increasing the rate of immunization, controlling sexually transmitted diseases, controlling the presence of toxic agents or radiation in the environment, improving occupational safety and health, preventing accidents, promoting water fluoridation and dental health, controlling infectious diseases, decreasing smoking, decreasing alcohol and drug abuse, improving nutrition, promoting physical fitness and exercise, and controlling stress and violent behavior. Great progress has been made in many of these areas. For example, the report *Health, United States, 1998* indicates that in general, the workplace is safer today than it was a decade ago. Between 1980 and 1993, the overall death rate from occupational injuries dropped 45 percent to 4.2 deaths per 100,000 workers.

For healthy adolescents and young adults (ages 15 to 24), the specific goal defined by the Public Health Service was a 20% reduction in deaths, with a special focus on motor vehicle injuries as well as alcohol and drug abuse. For adults (ages 25 to 64), the aim was 25% fewer deaths, with a concentration on heart attacks, strokes, and cancers. In the 1999 National Drug Control Strategy, the White House Office of National Drug Control Policy echoed the Congressional goal of reducing drug use by 50 percent in the coming decade.

Smoking is perhaps the best example of how individual behavior can have a direct impact on health. Today cigarette smoking is recognized as the most important single preventable cause of death in our society. It is responsible for more cancers and more cancer deaths than any other known agent; is a prime risk factor for heart and blood vessel disease, chronic bronchitis, and emphysema; and is a frequent cause of complications in pregnancies and of babies born prematurely, underweight, or with potentially fatal respiratory and cardiovascular problems.

Since the release of the Surgeon General's first report on smoking in 1964, the proportion of adult smokers has declined substantially, from 43% in 1965 to 30.5% in 1985. The rate of cigarette smoking among adults declined from 1974 to 1995, but rates of decline were greater among the more educated. Since 1965, more than 50 million people have quit smoking. Although the rate of adult smoking has decreased, children and teenagers are smoking more. Researchers have also noted a disturbing correlation between underage smoking of cigarettes and later use of cocaine and heroin. Although there is still much work to be done if we are to become a "smoke free society," it is heartening to note that public health and public education efforts—such as warnings on cigarette packages, bans on broadcast advertising, removal of billboards advertising cigarettes, and anti-drug youth campaigns in the media— have already had significant effects.

In 1997, the first leveling off of drug use since 1992 was found in eighth graders, with marijuana use in the past month declining to 10 percent. The percentage of eighth graders who drink alcohol or smoke cigarettes also decreased slightly in 1997. In 1994 and 1995, there were more than 142,000 cocaine-related emergency-room episodes per year, the highest number ever reported since these events were tracked starting in 1978. Illegal drugs present a serious threat to Americans who use these drugs. Addiction is a chronic, relapsing disease that changes the chemistry of the brain in harmful ways. The abuse of inhalants and solvents found in legal products like hair spray, paint thinner, and industrial cleaners—called "huffing" (through the mouth) or "sniffing" (through the nose)—has come to public attention in recent years. *The National Household Survey on Drug Abuse* discovered that among youngsters ages 12 to 17, this dangerous practice doubled between 1991 and 1996 from 10.3 percent to 21 percent. An alarming large number of children died the very first time they tried inhalants, which can also cause brain damage or injure other vital organs.

Another threat to public health comes from firearm injuries. Fortunately, the number of such assaults declined between 1993 and 1996. Nevertheless, excessive violence in our culture—as depicted in the mass media—may have contributed to the random shootings at Columbine High School in Littleton, Colorado, and elsewhere. The government and private citizens are rethinking how to reduce the fascination with violence so that America can become a safer, healthier place to live.

The "smart money" is on improving health care for everyone. Only recently did we realize that the gap between the "haves" and "have-nots" had a significant health component. One more reason to invest in education is that schooling produces better health.

In 1835, Alexis de Tocqueville, a French visitor to America, wrote, "In America, the passion for physical well-being is general." Today, as then, health and fitness are front-page items. But with the greater scientific and technological resources now available to us, we are in a far stronger position to make good health care available to everyone. With the greater technological threats to us as we approach the 21st century, the need to do so is more urgent than ever before. Comprehensive information about basic biology, preventative medicine, medical and surgical treatments, and related ethical and public policy issues can help you arm yourself with adequate knowledge to be healthy throughout life.

FOREWORD

Sandra Thurman, Director, Office of National AIDS Policy, The White House

A hundred years ago, an era was marked by discovery, invention, and the infinite possibilities of progress. Nothing piqued society's curiosity more than the mysterious workings of the human body. They poked and prodded, experimented with new remedies and discarded old ones, increased longevity and reduced death rates. But not even the most enterprising minds of the day could have dreamed of the advancements that would soon become our shared reality. Could they have envisioned that we would vaccinate millions of children against polio? Ward off the annoyance of allergy season with a single pill? Or give life to a heart that had stopped keeping time?

As we stand on the brink of a new millennium, the progress made during the last hundred years is indeed staggering. And we continue to push forward every minute of every day. We now exist in a working global community, blasting through cyber-space at the speed of light, sharing knowledge and up-to-the-minute technology. We are in a unique position to benefit from the world's rich fabric of traditional healing practices while continuing to explore advances in modern medicine. In the halls of our medical schools, tomorrow's healers are learning to appreciate the complexities of our whole person. We are not only keeping people alive, we are keeping them well.

Although we deserve to rejoice in our progress, we must also remember that our health remains a complex web. Our world changes with each step forward and we are continuously faced with new threats to our well-being. The air we breathe has become polluted, the water tainted, and new killers have emerged to challenge us in ways we are just beginning to understand. AIDS, in particular, continues to tighten its grip on America's most fragile communities, and place our next generation in jeopardy.

Facing these new challenges will require us to find inventive ways to stay healthy. We already know the dangers of alcohol, smoking and drug abuse. We also understand the benefits of early detection for illnesses like cancer and heart disease, two areas where scientists have made significant in-roads to treatment. We have become a well-informed society, and with that information comes a renewed emphasis on preventative care and a sense of personal responsibility to care for both ourselves and those who need our help.

Read. Re-read. Study. Explore the amazing working machine that is the human body. Share with your friends and your families what you have learned. It is up to all of us living together as a community to care for our well-being, and to continue working for a healthier quality of life.

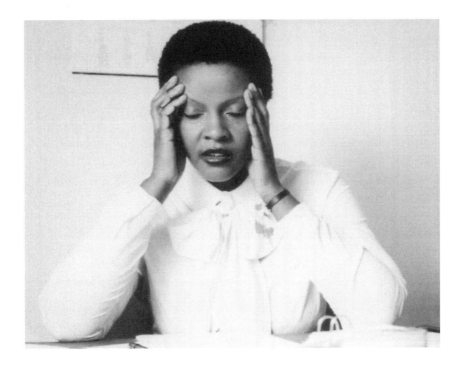

Almost everyone has felt the annoying pain of a headache: throbbing in the forehead, pressure at the temples, or the sensation that a metal band is tightening steadily around the skull. For many people, a headache is easy to cure. An aspirin or two, relaxation, or a good night's sleep banishes the pain completely.

For about 50 million people living in the United States, however, a headache is not just a temporary nuisance. These people suffer chronic headaches that either do not go away or recur repeatedly. Common remedies offer no relief, and the pain can be so severe that victims scream, cry, or pound their head against a wall. In self-portraits, these headache victims show devils drilling into their skull, bolts stinging their head, or lightning shooting from their eyes.

Parents afflicted with severe headaches sometimes cannot care for their children, hold a steady job, or participate in family and social events. Children of headache victims often must care for their parents instead of being cared for by them.

Many young people also suffer headaches. Statistics compiled by the National Headache Foundation show that the child of a person who gets migraine headaches—a severe, chronic ailment—stands a greater than 50% chance of developing such headaches, too, often before the age of 15. Less brutal headaches can also prove disruptive: each year headaches cause children and young adults to miss almost two million school days, according to findings issued by the National Center for Health Statistics.

Headaches have many different causes. A bite of ice cream can create sudden, sharp pain; anxiety over an upcoming school examination or sports tryout may cause the dull pounding of a tension headache. Sometimes the cause may be complex and obscure, and its cure can be costly or elusive.

Scientists have a great deal to learn about headaches. There is not even universal agreement about the exact causes of headache pain. Yet,

Each year headaches cause children and young adults to miss almost two million school days.

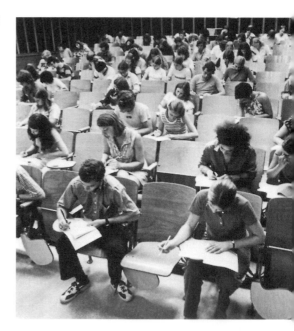

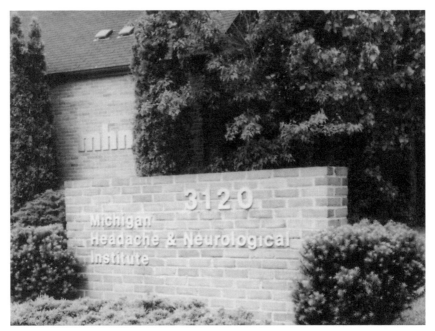

The Michigan Headache and Neurological Institute. In recent years, special clinics have offered new hope to headache sufferers.

because headaches are seldom life threatening, little money goes toward research on the subject. Furthermore, because no animals are known to get headaches, it is hard to design helpful laboratory experiments. Headache sufferers themselves remain a chief source of information about the ailment. Doctors and patients still await a major break-through in headache research.

But hope glimmers. In recent years, many new and at least par-tially effective treatments have been developed. Across the country, headache clinics offer help: For 9 out of 10 severe- or chronic-headache sufferers, the pain can be eased if not cured. For the rest, a new awareness on the part of friends and family—that the victim is not "faking it" or "making a big deal of nothing"—can make head-aches more tolerable.

Headaches remain among the most common and confusing of all ill-nesses. As a topic, headaches are highly interesting and have fascinated physicians and thinkers for thousands of years. This volume surveys what people of earlier times thought of headaches; describes the anatomy of the head and what makes it hurt; outlines the different types of headaches and their causes (insofar as they are known); explains what other ailments headaches may stem from or cause; discusses aspirin and other painkillers, including some nonchemical methods that can help; details the goings-on at a headache clinic; provides up-to-date information about how doctors work for better understanding and treatment of pain; and advises readers how to obtain further information on headaches and headache relief.

1

FROM MAGIC TO MEDICINE

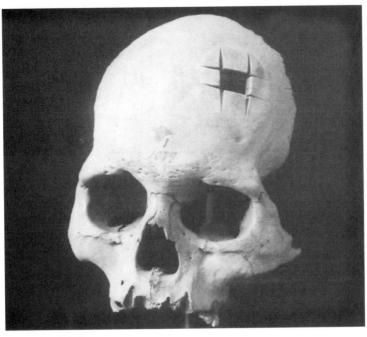

A trephined skull.

It seems that even before history was recorded, people suffered from headaches and searched for ways to cure them. Around the year 4000 B.C., in what is now France, Neolithic healers practiced a form of *trephination.* This procedure involved drilling or sawing holes in a headache sufferer's skull with sharpened stone tools, probably in order to let out the evil spirits they thought caused head pain and other illnesses. The bone pieces—called *rondelles* by modern scientists—removed from the patients' heads during the operation process may have been worn by the cured sufferers as amulets, charms meant to keep the departed spirits from returning. This primitive surgery was also performed by prehistoric peoples throughout Europe and in North and South America.

Knowledge about this surgery was gleaned in 1873 by French archaeologist M. Prunieres, who unearthed pierced skulls during his investigations of places where ancient people lived. Because some skulls showed signs of bone healing, it seems reasonable to assume that patients could survive for years after their surgery. And, although doctors today might fault the logic behind these ancient operations, the surgical method used was remarkably sophisticated. Indeed, contemporary surgeons sometimes trephine skulls to relieve pressure caused by bleeding or swelling.

The oldest-known written prescription for headaches was found by archaeologists on a clay tablet in the ruins of Sumer, a town in the Middle East that thrived about 5,000 years ago. The Sumerian cure called for a piece of goat's wool to be tied into 14 magic knots and wrapped around the sufferer's head while the healer prayed for the headache to rise into heaven. The headache's evil spirit was called Tiu; the incantation, or prayer, uttered against him was translated by English scholar Campbell Thompson in his book, *Devils and Evil Spirits of Babylon*. The prayer was said, in part, like this: "Headache roams over the desert, blowing like the wind. Flashing like lightning, it cuts off a man like a reed, a man who does not respect his god. It has struck him, breaking his heart; he staggers insanely."

Ancient as the prayer is, anyone who has suffered a bad headache will wince with recognition at the description of Tiu's wrath. Other tablets describe cases in which "his brow pains a man, and he vomits and is sick, his eyes being inflamed." This ailment was thought to result from a blow to the victim's head by an irate ghost. The Sumerians had a treatment: they burned human bones, soaked them in cedar oil, and then applied the potion, in the form of a poultice, to the victim's skin.

In about 2000 B.C., Egyptian physicians recorded some of their cases on papyrus, paper made from crushed reeds. One that survives tells how a doctor examining a case of head injury felt "a smash like the ridges in melted copper . . . and something inside that fluttered like the soft spot on a baby's skull." Another papyrus prescribes *ricinus*, a plant, as a cure for headaches. In 1929, W. R. Dawson translated the prescription in the English archaeological journal *Aegyptus:* "If the peel be soaked in water and applied to the sufferer's head, it will be cured at once, as though it had never suffered."

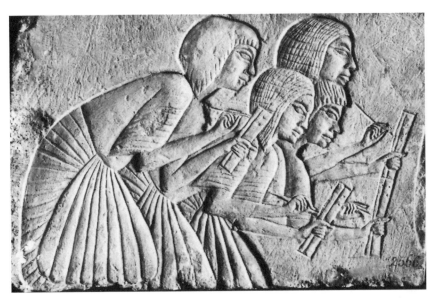

Ancient Egyptian physicians recorded some of their cases on papyrus, a paper made from crushed reeds. One such papyrus dating from about 2000 B.C. shows a prescription for a plant as a cure for headaches.

Later cultures also blamed headaches on superhuman forces. The ancient Greeks thought spirits called *keres* caused illnesses. According to the 4th-century B.C. philosopher Aristotle, the headache keres launched their invasions in the victim's head, where they caused pain. Several centuries later—and across the Mediterranean—the Romans thought their gods sent headaches to punish people who angered or insulted them. Thus, the English word *pain* derives from the Greek *poine,* meaning payment or penalty.

The first-line remedy for a Roman headache was a direct appeal to the offended god. Other approaches included knotting a hangman's rope around the victim's head, crowning him with a wreath made of an herb called fleabane, or encircling his neck with a red string of moss scraped from a statue. Roman philosopher Pliny the Elder, who lived in the 1st century A.D., believed this last method brought fast relief.

Early Christians also believed that prayer helped headaches. An 8th-century Irish monk wrote that the most effective means for banishing headaches was for the victim to pray to the eye of the prophet Isaiah, to the tongue of the wise king Solomon, to the mind of St. Benjamin, to the heart of St. Paul, and to the faith of Abraham. The victim was also advised to spit into his palm, trace the shape of a cross on his forehead,

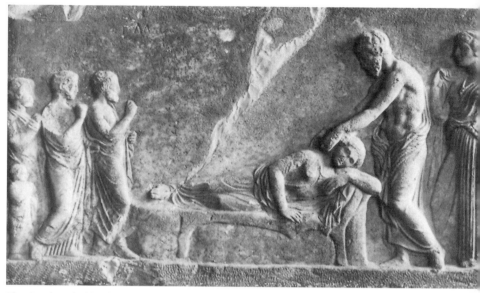

The Greek god of healing and medicine, Aesculapius, tending a patient. The ancient Greeks believed that spirits called keres *caused illnesses.*

and recite the Lord's Prayer three times, repeating the entire routine daily until the headache disappeared.

For centuries hair—because it grows from the head—has figured in many theories about the cause and cure of head pain. In the Middle Ages, Europeans guarded their hairbrushes, lest birds steal strands of hair for nests. Having one's hair woven into a bird's nest was considered a cause of headaches. Today, in many parts of the world, people still believe that hair plays a part in causing headaches. The Kai peoples of New Guinea, for example, believe an enemy can be given a headache if bits of his hair are stolen and burned with his food. In the Appalachian mountain regions of the United States, some people cut off their hair and bury it under a rock in the belief that the headache will thus be drawn out of the head.

The Roman method of making direct appeals to divinity also survives in the form of faith healing, practiced today by many religious people in the United States and elsewhere. Beliefs vary widely among faith healers and their followers, but most healers maintain that divine power is immediately available to those who believe in it and in God and that illnesses can be cured through this power if certain rituals are followed. For example, the healer may anoint the sick person with holy oil, then lay his or her hands on the sick person's body while praying intensely.

In eighth-century France, a cult dedicated to the healing properties of vultures arose. A curious manuscript, *Letter of the Vulture* (first translated into English in 1943), explains that a vulture's body could be used to cure headaches as long as the bird was killed with a sharp reed and its head bones wrapped in deerskin. The truly desperate sufferer might also try inhaling a concoction of vulture brains mixed with oil. Vulture cures are likely ancestors of a headache remedy commonly used on the American frontier, where headachy pioneers were advised to wear a dead buzzard's head on a cord around their neck.

The first known prescription for an oral headache remedy—that is, a remedy taken by mouth—was used in England in the ninth century. It consisted of elderberry-seed juice, cow brains, and goat droppings dissolved in vinegar. The vinegar cure survives to the present day in the form of such home remedies as tying a brown paper bag soaked in vinegar around the head or breathing the vapors of boiling vinegar.

By about the 13th century, herbal cures became popular in Europe. People wore garlands of dill, mugwort, and wormwood to relieve or prevent headaches. In Bohemia (now part of Czechoslovakia) during

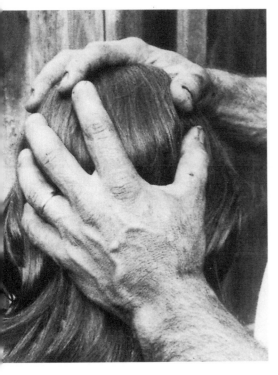

Many people believe that faith healing—healing through divine power—can cure headaches. An integral part of the healing process is the laying on of hands, shown here.

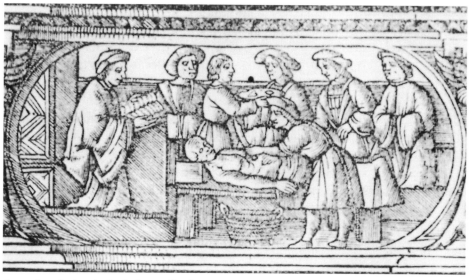

A woodcut depicts the herbal remedies that were popular headache treatments from the 13th through the 17th century.

the midsummer bonfire (a spectacle somewhat like U.S. Fourth of July fireworks), many Bohemians observed the flames through such a garland in the belief they would be headache free for the rest of the year.

By the 1600s, the list of herbal curatives included geraniums, roses, valerian, poppy seed, nutmeg, and walnuts. At about this time, one truly useful herb medication became known: *Atropa belladonna* leaves. If this plant was applied to the head, it seemed to relieve headache and to help people sleep. Later, this plant's extracts became the source of a medicine now used for eye and heart ailments: atropine.

During the same era, however, a more radical remedy for headache developed: exorcism. Jews and Christians alike believed that people who suffered violent headaches were possessed by Satan or his princes. To chase the demons away, clergymen and -women enacted complex rituals. One French nun was said to have been relieved of four devils, each ruling part of her head, after an exorcism that took four months.

Meanwhile, explorers of other frontiers came back from the New World (America) with remedies that did not require battles against evil spirits. One such "remedy" was tobacco, which was thought to cure headaches when sniffed. Another was castoretum, a preparation of beaver testes (the organ that produces sperm) soaked in alcohol. Native Americans used castoretum for headaches, but Europeans found it too repulsive. Castoretum was later found to contain salicylate, similar to the active ingredient contained in aspirin. This finding makes sense because salicylate comes from tree bark, which, along with marsh grasses, twigs, and roots, provides the beaver with its main source of nourishment.

The Cherokee tribes treated headaches with magic and the herb ginseng. The sufferer chewed ginseng while a medicine man rubbed the patient's head and sang: "The men have passed by, they have caused relief, / The wizards have passed by, they have caused relief. / Relief has been rubbed, they have caused relief. Sharp!" Then the medicine man sipped ginseng and water and blew on the sufferer's head four times.

In about 1710, the French physician Pierre Donis treated headaches with the "blister beetle." The beetles were killed, dried, powdered, mixed with yeast and vinegar to form a paste, and then applied to the head. When the resulting blisters broke, the headache drained away—or was supposed to. A hundred years later, this blister treatment using cantharis (known as Spanish fly) was still in use, along with other methods

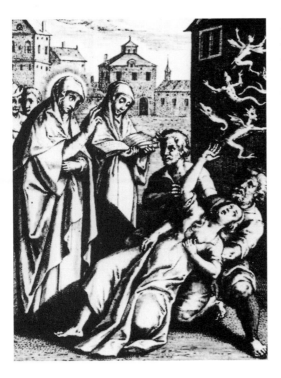

During the 17th century many people believed that headaches were a sign of demonic possession and could only be cured by exorcisms such as that shown here.

for drawing off "ill humours," such as draining blood from the body through incisions or with leeches.

In the 19th century, traveling European and American quacks—fakes who peddled cures from town to town—touted all sorts of bizarre headache cures. These ranged from worthless "eyeball vibrators" to potions that really relieved pain. The effective remedies were based on a number of 19th-century discoveries. In 1806, Frederick Serteurner, a German medical researcher, concocted the painkiller morphine from an extract of the opium poppy; in 1857 cocaine was isolated from the leaf of the South American coca plant. Alcohol, opium, morphine, cocaine, and codeine were major ingredients in dozens of 19th-century patent medicines that were supposed to cure "whatever ails you." These elixirs did sometimes cure headaches, but they also made addicts of so many of those who relied on them that in 1914 the U.S. Congress passed the Harrison Act, which controlled narcotic usage throughout the nation.

Headache sufferers still had hope, however. In 1830, salicylic acid—an effective nonnarcotic headache medicine made from willow bark—was discovered. Its synthetic counterpart, acetylsalicylic acid, was first

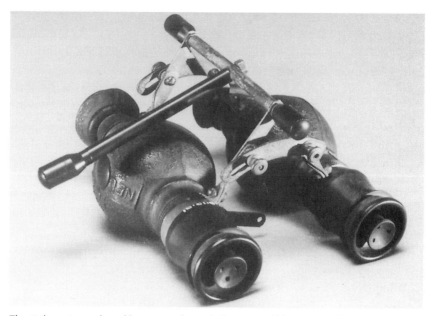

The 19th century ushered in an era of quack doctors and bizarre remedies for the relief of headache pain. This "eyeball vibrator," for example, was virtually useless.

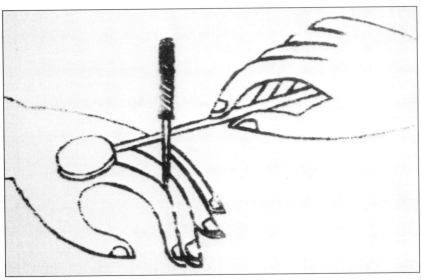

A page from an 18th-century manuscript shows the use of acupuncture, an ancient Chinese technique involving the use of small needles to stimulate nerves and block pain impulses.

sold as aspirin by the Bayer Drug Company in Germany. Bromo-Seltzer was another early aspirin-based cure for headaches.

Aspirin remains a common headache remedy to this day, but in the 20th century a number of new drugs for headache and other pain were also developed, including ibuprofen (found in the brands Advil and Nuprin) and acetaminophen (the main component in Tylenol). New ways of investigating headaches were tried as well, including a method devised by Dr. John Meyer, whose studies of blood flow in the brain provided doctors with new information about what chemically happens inside the head when a headache occurs.

Meanwhile, many headache sufferers rely on nondrug techniques, ancient and new. These cures include acupuncture (a technique in which small needles are placed in the skin to stimulate nerves and block pain impulses); biofeedback (learning to control pain and the mechanisms that cause it); hypnosis; relaxation and meditation; and innovative approaches such as music and laugh therapies.

Whatever methods are used against headaches, however, the risks of the treatment must always be weighed. A person who has an agonizing headache may be willing to "try anything," but doctors know that unwise cures often cause more harm than the disease. A "harmless" drug such as aspirin, for instance, can prove fatal for adults who swallow too many or for some children stricken with the flu. And regular use of powerful painkillers, such as codeine and morphine, can lessen their effectiveness and lead to addiction.

Unfortunately, the perfect headache cure has not yet been found. Thus, investigation into the causes of headaches continues, along with the ongoing search for safe, reliable headache relief.

2

THE HEAD—
INSIDE AND OUT

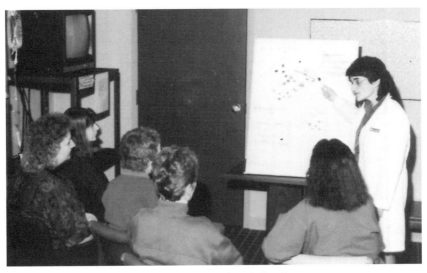

A nurse indicates pain-causing mechanisms to hospital patients.

The human head's many complex parts perform some of the body's most important functions. Four of the five sensory organs—the eyes, ears, nose, and tongue—are located in the head, along with structures in the inner ear that help maintain the body's equilibrium. The main requirements for life—air, water, and food—enter the body through specialized openings in the head, which also houses the organs that enable us to speak. In addition, the head serves as the repository for the brain. It encases and protects the brain and the upper spinal cord, which is located inside the skull.

Because the head consists of so many parts—each with a unique function and a distinct relationship to all the others—there are many different types of headache. And head pain can arise in a variety of places. Indeed, the quality of discomfort (whether the headache burns,

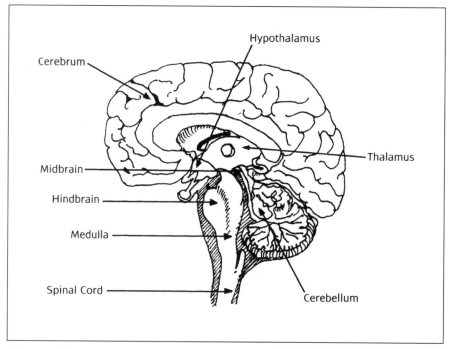

Figure 1: The Human Brain.

throbs, pierces, or pounds) and the intensity (from mild to excruciating) partly depend on what area of the head is sending pain messages.

A constant feature in all kinds of headaches, however, is pain, which is always produced and perceived by the same mechanism. Pain, the body's way of recognizing damage and then reacting to it, involves four processes or stages. The first, nociception, happens at the site of injury or irritation in *nociceptors*. These are special nerve cells that, like all nerve cells, are part of the nervous system, which itself has two main components: the central nervous system (made up of the brain and spinal cord) and the peripheral nervous system (the nerves that branch out to the rest of the body). When we bump our head, for example, painsensing nociceptors send pain signals along nerves from the bumped spot to the spinal cord and from there to the brain.

The next phase of pain occurs when chemicals at the injury site are released from the damaged area. Three of these chemicals are bradykinin, substance P, and prostaglandin. Bradykinin stimulates pain nerves, substance P causes them to remain stimulated, and prostaglandin helps transmit pain messages from nerve cell to nerve cell along the pathways to the brain.

It is impossible to grasp how these messages are relayed and how the body perceives pain without some knowledge of how the human brain works. The brain occupies the upper front half and the entire rear half of the inside of the skull. It is the central information processing department of the human body and consists of two types of tissue: white matter, consisting of nerve cells, and gray matter, the organ tissue of the brain itself.

The brain is protected by three membranes called the *dura mater,* the *arachnoid mater,* and the *pia mater.* Between the arachnoid and the pia is a layer of fluid (called cerebrospinal fluid) that circulates around the brain to cushion it and keep it moist; under normal conditions the brain is actually floating in this fluid.

From top to bottom, the brain is divided into the right- and left-sided cerebrum (the site of sensory, movement, and thought function); the similarly divided cerebellum (site of coordination and perception of space); the diencephalon or interbrain (where the thalamus and hypothalamus relay information from some sense organs, regulate the body's temperature, and coordinate some automatic nervous functions and the limbic system, a complex network of structures that control emotions); the midbrain (the relay station for sight and hearing information); the medulla (where nerves control breathing and influence heart action); and the spinal cord (a long stalklike structure that runs from the brain down inside the backbone, carrying nerve messages back and forth between the brain and the rest of the body).

In the brain, the pain signals reach the reticular formation, an area at the top of the spinal cord, and the thalamus, a relay station located in the base of the brain. From the thalamus, two kinds of signals are then sent: signals back down to the source of the pain, telling the pain to stop; and signals up to the cerebral cortex, the "thinking" part of the brain where the pain is actually perceived.

The stop-pain system works like this: substance P, a protein that causes pain nerves to remain active once they have been stimulated, enables pain messages to be transmitted from nerve to nerve along the nervous system. Once the signals reach the brain, the brain releases "stop" chemicals—the neurotransmitters serotonin and norepinephrine. These two chemicals trigger the release of endorphins (natural morphinelike substances that slow down the release of substance P)

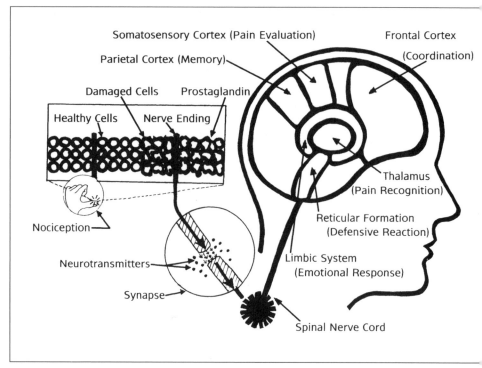

Figure 2: The Path of Pain.

and GABA (gamma-aminobutyric acid, a chemical that lowers sensitivity in the nerve cells).

As it travels to the cerebral cortex, the pain signal passes through the limbic system, the part of the interbrain that controls emotions. Our shout of pain, our tears, or our feelings of fear—the expressions of suffering—originate here and form the third phase of the cycle.

Even as these events occur, the rest of the body feels the effect of the pain messages, which, like the brain's stop messages, actually consist of potent chemicals called neurotransmitters. Four major ones are acetylcholine, dopamine, epinephrine, and norepinephrine. They increase the heart rate and blood pressure and send more sugar into the blood—all part of a reaction known as fight or flight, the body's automatic preparations to handle danger, conflict, pain, or another threat by moving determinedly either toward or away from the threat.

Once the pain messages reach the cerebral cortex, the fourth phase of pain occurs. This is the sufferer's reaction, the way he or she tends to adapt to pain. For example, one person may retreat into a dark room, whereas another will seek the distraction of activity. So-called pain be-havior may be influenced by many factors: cultural habits, the victim's memory of previous experiences, and anxiety or fear all shape individual responses to pain and individual levels of tolerance.

Although the brain itself enables us to perceive pain, it is not sensitive to it. Brain tissue has no nociceptors and thus cannot feel any damage that may occur to it. For this reason some kinds of brain surgery do not require the use of anesthesia.

Other components of the head—the bones, for example—are well supplied with nociceptors and can produce pain messages. The bones in the head account for the shape of the face and also shield the brain from damage. Together these bones make up the skull, a rigid structure that has two sections: the cranium and the facial bones. The cranium consists of eight bones fused together: the two parietal bones, the occipital bone, the two temporal bones (the body's hardest bones), the spheroid and ethmoid bones, and the frontal bone.

The bones of the face are also fused, except for one joint—the tem-poromandibular joint—that allows jaw movement for speaking and eating. Major facial bones include the mandible (lower jaw) and the maxilla (upper jaw), in which the teeth are firmly rooted. Other main facial bones include the cheek and nose bones, the lacrimal (eye-socket) bones, and the palatine bones that form the roof of the mouth. Several frontal bones contain hollow spaces, called sinuses, that open into the nasal passages.

The bones of the upper spinal column—beginning at the base of the skull—are called the cervical vertebrae. They enclose and protect the spinal cord; the two topmost bones of the spinal column also help hold up the head and allow it to turn and flex.

The bones of the head may cause pain directly when they are bruised or fractured or when their cells are invaded by infection or tumor. The relative rigidity of head bones does not allow their contents enough room to expand when structures inside the skull swell because of illness or injury, and the resulting pressure can create pain. Unlikely as it may seem, the neck is a common source of headaches because branches of the trigeminal nerve, a main nerve in the head, also extend into the neck. Thus injury or disease in the upper neck can cause headaches felt in the eye or forehead.

The muscles of the head and neck are divided into three groups. The muscles used for facial expression are responsible for movements of the mouth, cheeks, forehead, and of the skin around the eyes. Muscles of

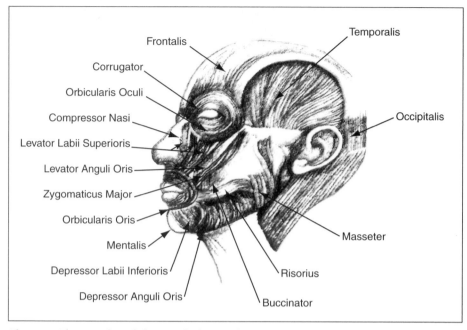

Figure 3: The Muscles of the Head. *The muscles of the head can cause headache pain if they are infected, injured, or damaged by tumor.*

mastication are responsible for jaw movement, the movement of the tongue, and some movements involved in swallowing. Neck muscles include the anterior (front) and posterior (back) neck muscles and the sternocleidomastoid and trapezius muscles that run along its sides.

When the muscles of the head and neck are injured or when they are damaged by infection or tumor, headaches can result. At one time, chronic tension headaches were thought to be caused by constant tensing of these muscles. Some studies suggest, however, that sufferers of chronic tension headaches often have no more muscle tenseness than nonsufferers. But the matter may not be quite so simple. In *Freedom from Headaches,* by Joel Saper and Kenneth R. Magee, Dr. Seymour Diamond, who heads the Diamond Headache Clinic in Chicago, says that at least 50% of the people his clinic treats each year who are afflicted with daily tension headaches may also suffer from emotional depression.

Blood vessels located in the brain and scalp are another source of headache pain. When they are disturbed or stretched, their special pain-sensing cells, called stretch receptors, protest vigorously. Causes of headaches arising from this occurrence range from acute infection

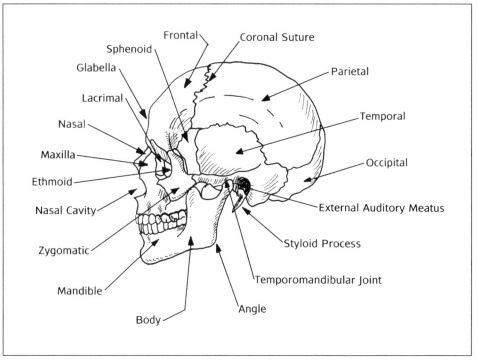

Figure 4: The Bones of the Skull. *The bones of the head may cause headache pain when they are bruised or fractured or when they are invaded by tumor or infection.*

or high blood pressure to simply drinking too much coffee. When a brain tumor causes a headache—one of the rarer causes of head pain—it does so by pressing on blood vessels and activating their stretch receptors.

Another source of headache is the eye, a complex structure resting in the bony eye-socket and controlled by six muscles that allow it to move. Information from the eye travels along the optic nerve to a part of the brain called the visual cortex. The eye and the areas near it are rich in muscles, sensory nerves, and pain receptors. All these provide many opportunities for headaches to develop. The glare of the sun or a long period of reading or staring at the TV can cause a nonthreatening but painful headache. More serious developments in the eye, such as tumor, nerve injury, or infection, may also cause head pain.

Some headaches originate in the ear, which consists of three parts: the outer ear, ending at the tympanic membrane or eardrum; the middle ear, where three small bones called the hammer, anvil, and stirrup transmit sound vibrations inward; and the inner ear, where sound is translated into nerve impulses for transmission via the cochlear nerve to the brain. The inner ear also contains three fluid-filled canals that maintain our balance. When we shift position, fluid in the canals moves, sending nerve impulses to the brain, which help maintain equilibrium and prevent dizziness. Like the eye, the ear is rich in potential sources of pain. Headaches arising from the ear may come from tumor, injury, or infection, or from much less serious causes, such as exposure to loud or persistent noise.

In the area of the mouth and nose, structures that can cause headache include the teeth (infection, injury, incorrect position), the jaw muscles (tenseness), and the sinuses, the hollows in facial bones near the nose. The sinuses usually drain into the nasal passages, but if they are blocked—for example, by infection or by swelling from allergies—pressure from the obstruction can cause a sinus headache.

The final cause of headaches is the nerves; carriers of pain messages, they can also create them. Pain arising from a nerve is called neuralgia and may be caused by injury, infection, pressure (from the swelling of a tumor or from scar tissue, for instance), or chronic irritation from pain originating somewhere else.

Although the head is a complex and important part of the body, most of its pains result in ordinary headaches that pose no danger in themselves and hint at no more serious condition elsewhere in the body. But, as everyone knows, ordinary headaches are painful and troublesome enough, and, as such, merit discussion.

3

OH, MY HEAD!

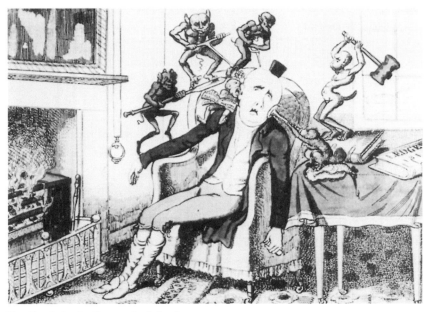

The Headache *by George Cruikshank.*

Why do some generally healthy people get more headaches than other people do? One explanation probably lies in their genetic makeup: they may inherit genes for more numerous and more effective neurotransmitters than others. As headache researcher Dr. Joel Saper pointed out in a 1987 interview in *Newsweek*, "Headache is perhaps only the tip of a biological iceberg. There may be a basic . . . problem that's the common denominator in family trees."

Most researchers think the brain's internal pain-control mechanisms play a role in regulating headache frequency and severity. It also seems that people who are usually happy tend to have fewer headaches than unhappy people. In an article that appeared in the 1987 National Headache Foundation newsletter, Dr. Seymour Diamond suggested that depression may also play an important—though, as yet, mysterious—part in causing headaches. The question remains open to debate, however. After all, it may be their tendency to suffer headaches that affects the temperament of many victims. In any case, headache causes and symptoms overlap to a confusing degree, often frustrating physicians and headache sufferers alike.

Many ordinary headaches, however, can be traced to causes experienced by most of us at one time or another. Among the most common of these is the tension headache.

TENSION HEADACHE

When a tension headache hits, the sufferer often feels a dull, constant, heavy, tight, or pressing pain on both sides of the head and also, in some cases, in the neck. Episodes of stabbing pain also occur, and the sufferer may sink into depression, sadness, or anxiety. Some people suffer only occasional tension headaches and are helped by mild pain relievers such as aspirin. Others, however, are chronically besieged and gain scant relief from standard medications. Still others have tension headaches that last all day long, for months, or even years.

Tension headaches can arise during anxious times: before a medical or dental procedure, an important school examination, or a social event. People with uneven teeth may get tension headaches from chronic strain on their jaw muscle. Eyestrain, loud noise, bright lights, a stuffy room, or a stiff neck may also bring on tension headaches in susceptible persons; still others appear to get them frequently for no apparent reason.

Exactly what makes a person prone to tension headache is still under investigation, as are the specific physical events that trigger the headache and cause the pain. Muscle tension is thought to be a culprit in some sufferers. Most psychological tests disclose no personality difference between sufferers and the rest of the population. People who frequently suffer tension headaches are sometimes bracketed with victims of other diseases, such as ulcers and chronic diarrhea, that are often labeled as psychosomatic—related to or caused by a person's mental or emotional state. But emotions are not believed to be the whole answer to the cause of tension headaches.

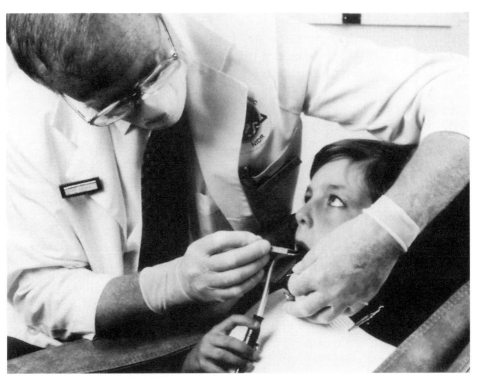

Tension headaches often arise during anxiety-provoking situations. The fear that often accompanies a trip to the dentist, for example, can lead to one of these painful episodes.

Some clues to tension headaches surfaced in research in biochemistry, the study of chemical activity in living creatures. In a test conducted in 1980 and reported in the medical journal *Pain,* histamine—a powerful blood vessel dilator—was given to some people who suffered chronic tension headaches and to some who did not. Half the chronic-headache group experienced severe headaches from histamine, whereas practically none of those who were not chronic-headache victims felt any negative effects. In another experiment, reported in 1981 in the journal *Headache,* the blood content of serotonin—one of the body's pain-regulating substances—was found to be significantly lower in headache sufferers than in those who were usually headache free.

A great deal remains to be learned about all the elements that contribute to tension headaches, but it is known that lessening stress and anxiety can help prevent them. If the headaches occur only once in a while, two aspirin tablets and a brief period of rest may help dispel them. If tension headaches are frequent or disabling, however, a physician's program for prevention and relief may include relaxation exercises, muscle-relaxing drugs such as diazepam (Valium), and hypnotism.

If such therapy fails, the physician may recommend the antidepressant drugs amitriptyline (Elavil) or imipramine (Tofranil). These drugs also improve the condition of patients who are not depressed, apparently by helping the body regulate its own serotonin levels. An early study by Dr. J. W. Lance, in Australia, showed that patients who used these drugs recovered from tension headaches more than 50% of the time. Unfortunately, these drugs have side effects. Patients are often afflicted with drowsiness, trembling, dry mouth, and blurred vision and have trouble urinating. Consequently, doctors prescribe these drugs only when other methods have failed and even then carefully supervise the patients' use of them.

VASCULAR HEADACHE

Another common headache is vascular headache, caused by a disturbance or swelling of blood vessels in the head. Unlike most other headaches, vascular headaches are characterized by pounding; the sufferer may feel each heartbeat as a painful "thud" in the skull. The mechanism by which a vascular headache begins is not fully known, though some physicians think it starts when serotonin released from nerve cells enters the blood vessels in the brain. The presence of serotonin in the blood vessels, along with the presence of bradykinin, the potent pain-producing substance, makes them extrasensitive to pain. At the same time the shortage of serotonin in the nervous system enables pain impulses to pass through the nerve cells to the brain with unusual ease.

What initially triggers a vascular headache? One possible cause is food: hot dogs, bacon, ham, salami, and some other artificially preserved foods contain nitrites, which are chemicals added during processing to give the appearance of a uniform color. Nitrates, which are known to dilate blood vessels, are frequently added to foods in a concentration of only 50 to 130 parts per million, but this dosage is enough to affect persons who are sensitive to them.

Another common food additive, monosodium glutamate (MSG), also dilates blood vessels and causes headaches in people sensitive to the substance, especially if they ingest it on an empty stomach. MSG is often used as a food additive to heighten the taste of foods—particularly Chinese food. The headache it produces is sometimes called the "Chinese restaurant syndrome."

SIDE EFFECTS AND DANGERS OF ASPIRIN USE

Many people think of aspirin as a cure-all and take it for relief from headache, fever, arthritis pain, and other ailments. But this useful remedy has side effects, ranging from mild discomforts, such as an irritated stomach lining, to severe disorders, such as allergic shock. For certain people the dangers of aspirin are especially great. Asthma sufferers may be allergic to the drug and should use it only with caution. Pregnant women can suffer hemorrhaging after taking aspirin. If taken in strong doses, the drug can also endanger young children.

One potential side effect of aspirin use that is of particular concern is Reye's syndrome. First recognized as a disease in 1963 by Australian pathologist R. Douglas Reye, Reye's syndrome is a childhood ailment that strikes during the winter months, usually following the onset of a common childhood infection such as influenza or chicken pox. Just when the child appears to be recovering from the infection, a new array of symptoms may strike, including persistent and severe vomiting, drowsiness, lack of interest in normally enjoyable activities, and delirium. In some extreme cases, the child may lapse into a coma. All these symptoms indicate Reye's syndrome, a disease that if left unattended can prove fatal.

Scientists are as yet unsure about the exact cause of the disease, but they suspect a link between Reye's syndrome and the use of aspirin during a viral illness. Studies have shown that children given an aspirin substitute during their illness were far less likely to develop Reye's syndrome than were children treated with aspirin. Consequently, doctors caution parents not to give their children aspirin during a viral illness. Acetaminophen or another effective aspirin substitute poses far less risk. Indeed, many physicians maintain that children under 16 should completely avoid aspirin under all circumstances and instead take acetaminophen for pain and fever relief.

For most people, acetaminophen is an ideal aspirin substitute because it is less irritating to the stomach and is equally effective in treating most of the same illnesses. However, asthma sufferers should be aware that acetaminophen, like aspirin, can cause an allergic reaction and shock. In addition, if taken in quantities that exceed the recommended dosage, acetaminophen can cause liver damage.

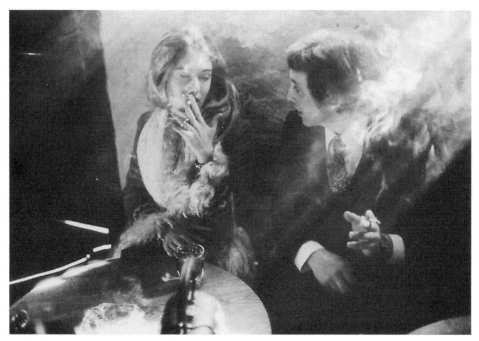

Both alcohol and nicotine can lead to vascular headaches, which are caused by a disturbance or swelling of the blood vessels in the head.

Yet another potent vessel dilator is alcohol. Even moderate drinking can cause headaches in persons sensitive to trace elements (tiny amounts of chemicals) in red wine, beer, and—to a lesser degree—in other alcoholic drinks. The by-products of alcohol digestion (acetaldehyde and acetate) also widen blood vessels, which is another reason why a bad headache accompanies a hangover.

Hunger can also produce a headache because lowered blood sugar—one result of going for an extended period of time without eating—causes fatty acids to be released into the bloodstream. Consequently, blood vessels widen and a dull, pounding head pain results. People who often fall prey to such headaches can stave off attacks by eating four to six small low-sugar meals per day.

"Rebound" headaches, often dull and pounding, begin when the blood vessels are constricted by substances such as caffeine (found in coffee, tea, colas, and some over-the-counter [OTC] pain relievers); nicotine (the primary drug found in cigarettes); and some prescribed medications. Chronic use of these substances causes the vessels to be partly constricted all the time; when the user fails to take the substance—for instance, when someone who usually drinks a lot of coffee does not drink the usual amount—the vessels "rebound" to a painfully dilated state. These headaches can be prevented if the sufferer gradually decreases his or her intake of the offending substance.

Even exercise can cause a headache. Many young people, in fact, are tempted to give up because the exertion gives them such terrible head pain. This is because exercise raises the pulse rate and blood pressure and dilates the arteries, the vessels that carry blood from the heart to the body's tissues. People who suffer exercise headaches do so because their small vessels do not widen sufficiently to accept the increased blood flow. The blood backs up slightly, widening the larger vessels and causing pain. Luckily, the problem is often treatable with drugs that, if taken before a workout, prevent excessive vessel dilation and stop the pain.

Headaches can also result from coughing, sneezing, bending, or straining—activities that temporarily raise the blood pressure and

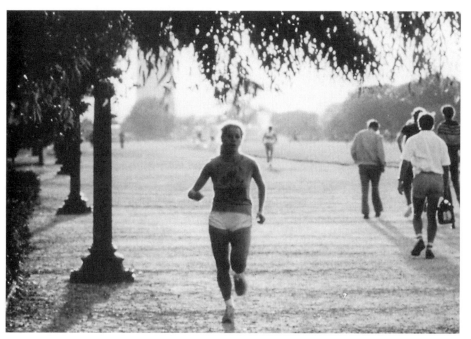

Some people experience headache pain while exercising because their blood vessels are not wide enough to facilitate the increased blood flow that accompanies exercise.

thus widen the vessels in the brain. Men are victimized by this pain four times more often than women, though no one knows why. People prone to this sort of headache should be checked by a physician because it can indicate other serious problems such as fluid blockage in the brain. The condition almost always proves harmless, however. In a study of 103 people with "cough headache," only 10 had abnormalities that needed treatment, and in 73 the headache eventually went away by itself.

CLUSTER HEADACHE

A severe type of headache related to blood vessel disturbance is the cluster headache, also called "macho" headache because 85% of its victims are men, usually smokers, and alcohol use may trigger attacks. Cluster headaches tend to strike their victims first during the teen years. About 1 in 40 people—a total of some 5 million Americans—suffer this painful ailment.

Cluster headaches occur in brief episodes, sometimes a dozen or more a day. These can be so painful that victims pound their head against walls or roll on the floor in anguish. The pain, along with tearing eyes and a runny or blocked nose, may recur every day or night, for weeks, months, or even years. Often, the eye on the affected side becomes bloodshot and its pupil constricts during an attack. The vision may blur, the forehead sweats, the scalp feels tender, and hivelike lumps rise on the inside of the mouth.

The timing of cluster headaches often resemble that of an internal clock, striking at the same time each day and night. In his book *Migraine and Other Headaches,* Dr. James W. Lance reports: "A patient of mine who travels across Australia from Perth to Sydney (a 2,000 mile journey with a two hour change in time zones) told me that his cluster headache continued to wake him from sleep on Perth time until he adjusted his biological rhythms, when his headaches woke him at the same hour on Sydney time!"

At present no known cure exists for cluster headaches, but one effective way to gain relief is to breathe pure oxygen until the pain goes away—which it does within a few minutes in 80% of the cases. Some people keep oxygen tanks at home for this purpose. Steroids, such as prednisone, are effective preventatives. These drugs help about 75% of all patients, but because steroids cause strong and even hazardous side effects—including emotional disturbances, ulcers, increased blood pressure, blood clots, and facial swelling—they should not be used for long periods of time. Lithium carbonate, a medicine used to treat some forms of mental illness, also prevents some cluster headaches, but it, too, has potent side effects, such as hair loss, dizziness, weakness, and vomiting. People afflicted with frequent cluster headaches—a condition called *chronic paroxysmal hemicrania*—sometimes respond to indomethacin (Indocin), a drug used to treat pains in the joints.

TIC DOULOUREUX

Another headache that occurs in episodes is *tic douloureux* (French for "painful spasm"), a brief but severe stabbing pain that assails the gums, cheek, or chin when triggered by air moving against the cheek. It is caused not by blood vessel disturbance but by a change in the nerve impulse running along the trigeminal nerve (and therefore is also called trigeminal neuralgia). Why the nerve becomes sensitive in some people is not fully understood. Tic douloureux attacks women twice as often as men and usually surfaces after the victim reaches her forties. Some patients are helped by drugs ordinarily used to fight epilepsy, such as carbamazepine (Tegretol), or by antispasm drugs, such as baclofen (Lioresal). A few victims need surgery (to remove tissue that may be pressing on the trigeminal nerve) before they can be relieved of their misery.

SECONDARY HEADACHES

Secondary headaches result from injury or illness. The most common headaches of this sort are symptoms of mild disorders—the flu, for instance. Another of the common "secondaries" is sinus headache. This malady begins when one of the hollows in the victim's facial bones becomes blocked by tissues swollen from an allergy or infection. The sinus's usual outlet into the nasal passage does not drain properly, and pressure builds. This irritates nerve branches in the face and head, and pain arises. Treatment generally includes antibiotics (if infection is to blame); antihistamines (if allergy is the cause); and—to allow free drainage—decongestants (medications that shrink tissue). On a rare occasion, a physician may recommend surgery to open the blocked sinus.

A secondary headache can stem from an infected tooth because of a process, called "referred pain," whereby the irritation is passed along to nerves not directly in contact with the tooth. The ice cream headache—sudden pain that happens after biting into ice cream—is also caused by referred pain. In this instance it travels from the roof of the mouth to the trigeminal nerve.

As we have already seen, eye problems—ranging from simple strain to infection and tumor—can also cause headaches. Stronger reading light, rest periods during long study sessions, and regular eye examinations—with a prescription for corrective lenses if needed—commonly solve or prevent simple, uncomplicated eye-related headaches.

The common "whiplash" injury, caused by a sudden-stop car accident, and the degenerative bone disease rheumatoid arthritis also account for secondary headaches.

Finally, the wide category of common, nondangerous but troublesome headaches includes some that cannot be traced to any physical root: nothing is wrong with the body, yet it suffers pain. Some such headaches may result from physical malfunctions too subtle for current medical science to find. Others may be "conversion headaches,"

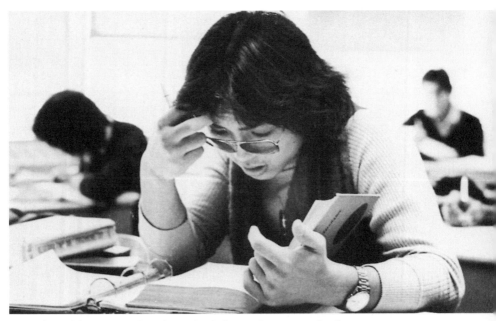

Eyestrain and the pressure that often exists before an important school exam are two more sources of tension headaches.

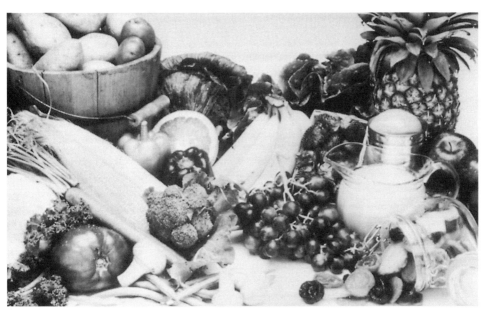

Eating healthy foods and refraining from those that bring on headache is just one of the measures people can take to avoid this condition.

that is, the products of emotional pain—such as grief, guilt, or anger—that are translated into physical pain in ways not yet fully understood.

This does not mean that a person who claims to have such a headache is faking it. Emotional pain, no less than primary physical pain, merits treatment. Once a physician has ruled out all plausible physical causes for chronic headaches, a psychologist or psychiatrist may be able to help the patient by treating the underlying emotional causes that trigger the physical pain and thus reduce the frequency and severity of conversion headaches.

The headache is a common ailment with a bewildering number of possible causes. We can improve our chances of avoiding ordinary headaches by refraining from alcohol, cigarettes, caffeine, and any food or foods to which we may be sensitive. A yearly eye examination and medical check-up as well as regular trips to the dentist will help protect us from several types of headache. And a balanced diet, regular exercise, and regular sleep habits, all of which keep us fit, also make us less vulnerable to headaches.

In spite of these efforts, an occasional headache is something we all experience. Usually a couple of aspirin and perhaps a brief rest relieve this temporary discomfort. Those who are allergic to aspirin should instead consult their physician for aspirin-free pain-relief alternatives.

Pain is not the only consequence of headaches. They also sap our time and savings, especially because an effective remedy can be hard to find. There is much each of us needs to know about aspirin and other medications: what they are made of, how they work, and what their side effects are.

4

THE $500-MILLION
HEADACHE

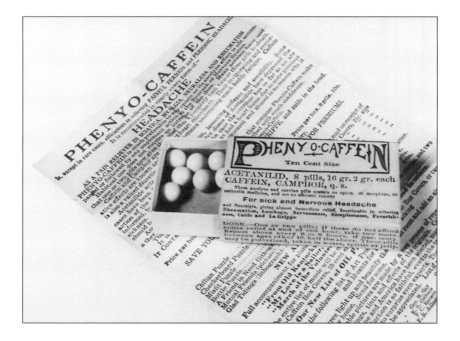

M any people view headaches as a nuisance rather than an illness.
Consequently, a headache victim does not get much sympathy:
missing school or work because of a headache is generally
frowned upon, for instance, whereas absence due to a stomachache
seems more legitimate.

According to neurologist David Rosenfield, "A person with his arm
in a sling will get more sympathy than someone who suffers headaches
every day." Yet headaches are responsible for an enormous amount of
pain and disruption in the lives of all kinds of people of all ages.

Children, once thought immune to headaches, are now known to
suffer significantly from them: 20% of all children get serious tension

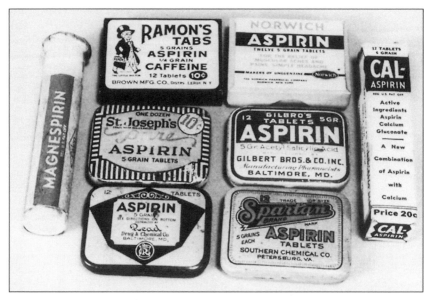

A selection of patent medicines once used as headache treatments. It is estimated that headache sufferers spend over $500 million each year in the United States alone in an effort to combat pain.

or other kinds of headaches, and 40% of migraine-headache victims suffer their first attack before the age of 15.

The 50 million Americans who suffer from chronic headaches, spend more than $500 million on OTC pain-relief preparations such as aspirin, acetaminophen, and ibuprofen. In addition, American businesses lose billions of dollars per year in costs incurred as a result of headache-related absenteeism and by business-paid medical expenses for employees who undergo headache treatments.

In short, headaches exact a heavy toll. In part, this is because head pain differs from all other pain. Though felt primarily in the head, it seems to affect every other part of the body. It also depletes the sufferer's energy and can hurtle him or her into a state of depression and helplessness. A bad headache seems to strike at the very essence of a person, at the center of his or her consciousness. Some desperate victims contemplate suicide.

So extreme a measure can seem to them the only solution to an ailment that, in many instances, can neither be explained nor cured. Current research has yielded answers for some headache sufferers, but others suffer and search for relief, usually in vain. For this reason headache victims are especially vulnerable to quackery such as "miracle" headache cures sold through magazine ads. Fake cures range from crystals that supposedly attract healing powers of the universe to "secret" potions, powders, and pills said to purify the blood or draw off toxic substances.

The only real power these "secret miracle cures" possess is emptying the wallets and pocketbooks of innocent sufferers, who will try anything in the hope of relieving their misery. Fakes who capitalize on these people's misery are not only dishonest but dangerous, because the false hope offered by phony cures may delay a necessary visit to a reputable practitioner.

Yet, the matter is not so easily settled. There are headache sufferers who gain some relief from medically worthless cures, or placebos. This term (a Latin word meaning "I will please") describes medications, usually in pill form, that contain no active ingredient. Placebos are often prescribed by physicians who suspect their patient's pain is psychological rather physiological.

About 40% of the patients who receive placebos for headaches report that the "medicine" relieves their pain partially or completely. A study of 188 headache sufferers by Dr. James Couch of Southern Illinois University Medical School found more than half the patients experienced improvement after receiving a placebo. As Couch said in an interview with *Newsweek* published in 1987, "Any time a patient walks into the office of a competent physician and is diagnosed, there's a 63% chance he'll get significantly better." Exactly how and why placebos work is not entirely understood, however.

PAIN RELIEF

Drugs that legitimately act to relieve headache pain—pills that contain chemically active ingredients—fall into three categories: analgesics, which lessen sensations of pain; mood-altering drugs; and drugs that directly combat the cause of the headache.

The simplest, least costly, and most frequently used analgesic for headache sufferers is aspirin. It is also one of the oldest. A crude form of the drug, willow bark tea, had long been in use by 1830, when the active ingredient in the bark, salicylic acid, was identified and isolated. Then, as mentioned in Chapter 1, the Bayer Company promptly created a synthetic form of the chemical, acetylsalicylic acid, and marketed it as aspirin. But it was not until 1982 that scientists Sune Bergstrom, Bengt Samuelsson, and John Vane learned how aspirin

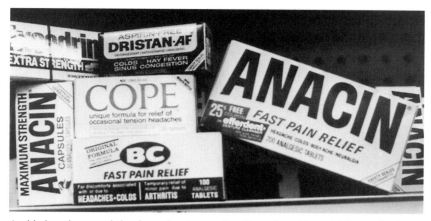

Aspirin is a cheap and simple analgesic, or pain reliever. But although it is an effective treatment for headache, it is also a stomach irritant and an anticoagulant and therefore should be used with caution.

works. It interferes with prostaglandin, a substance produced by the body when its tissues are damaged. This reaction won its discoverers the Nobel Prize in medicine.

Aspirin is taken by an estimated 42 million Americans each week. But this simple, effective remedy is not entirely harmless, and there are many people who must avoid it. Aspirin is a powerful anticoagulant (blood thinner) and so should not be used at all by hemophiliacs (people whose blood does not clot properly) or by those who take prescribed blood thinners. Aspirin can irritate the stomach lining and so should be avoided by people with stomach ulcers. It can also interfere with the absorption of other medications. In addition, about 1% of the population is allergic to aspirin. For these people, aspirin can cause rashes, breathing difficulties, or shock. Up to 20% of people afflicted with asthma (a respiratory condition resulting in attacks characterized by tightening in the chest, difficulty breathing, and wheezing) may be allergic to aspirin, so they should use it with extreme caution and only under the supervision of their physician.

Even people who can take aspirin safely should limit their dosages. The normal dosage for an adult or young person of adult weight is 1 or 2 300–325 mg tablets taken every 4 to 6 hours. The Food and Drug Administration's Advisory Review Panel estimates that a normal dose of aspirin may equal the painkilling power of an equivalent dose of a narcotic such as codeine. The FDA recommends that no more than 650 mg

AURAL DISTURBANCES

Migraine can lead to a wide variety of visual distortions—usually referred to as visual aura—that can be quite vivid and alarming. In the past, when little was understood about headaches or their symptoms, visual aura was often attributed to far-fetched causes. Sometimes the devil was blamed; sometimes the patient was thought to be a lunatic; and sometimes auras were interpreted as mystical visions. Contemporary scientists propose that many of these otherworldly experiences can be attributed to simple biological, chemical, or physical causes—epilepsy, accidental drug overdose or poisoning, psychosis, and migraine aura.

In *Migraine,* Dr. Oliver Sacks, a noted British neurologist and science writer, discusses the case of Hildegard of Bingen (1098–1180), a nun celebrated for the numerous visions she experienced. In one well-known episode, Hildegard believed she witnessed stars falling from the heavens into the ocean. She described seeing "a great star most splendid and beautiful, and with it an exceeding multitude of falling stars with which the star followed southwards."

Sacks maintains that the nun was a migraine sufferer who experienced visual distortions brought about by chemical changes within her brain. Sacks concedes that usually scientists can only speculate as to whether or not some person in the past suffered from a particular ailment; but, he argues, in the case of Hildegard of Bingen, the evidence is conclusive.

Today migraine sufferers understand the reasons for their aural disturbances and rarely accept outlandish explanations. Yet the intensity of the disturbances is no less real than in earlier times, and the episodes can be equally frightening. Among the many cases Sacks cites is that of a contemporary physician who suffers from auras that fill him with fear because without warning they cause him to witness changes that seem to transfigure the face of some patients. The physician himself describes a typical experience in harrowing terms: "I suddenly 'realize'—*part of the patient's face is missing:* part of their nose, or their cheek, or perhaps the left ear . . . a sense of horror, of the impossible, steals over me."

Thus, although migraine auras are better understood today than in the past, they can still overwhelm those who suffer from them. Worse, the sufferer may find little sympathy and understanding from those around him—friends, family, co-workers—who may wrongly attribute the symptoms to a serious mental illness, the same false assumption often made many centuries ago.

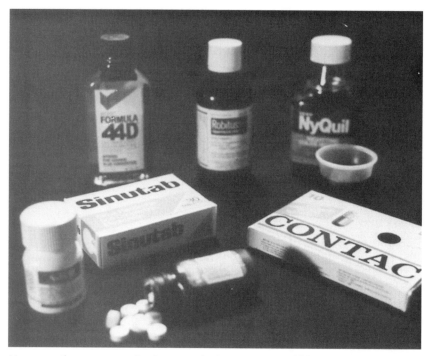

Many over-the-counter medications contain decongestants, which are often poorly absorbed by the body and may raise heart rate and blood pressure to dangerous levels.

aspirin be taken 4 times per day—400–500 mg for 9–12-year-olds—in order to avoid a painful stomach upset or even serious bleeding.

Young people, in particular, should be aware of the dangers of aspirin. In fact, they may run a higher risk of experiencing side effects, including Reye's syndrome, a potentially fatal complication of some viral illnesses such as chicken pox and the flu. For this reason the American Academy of Pediatrics recommends that children and young adults abstain from aspirin when suffering or recovering from viral illnesses. In addition, some physicians advise that people under the age of 16 should not take aspirin at all. Instead, they can use acetaminophen, a similar drug.

Acetaminophen—sold under the brand names Datril, Tylenol, and Liquiprin—works like aspirin against pain and fever but may be less irritating to the stomach. The usual dosage of acetaminophen is the same as that of aspirin. Only the recommended dosage should be taken in order to avoid potential damage to the liver.

Many other OTC medicines promise fast relief of headaches. Often these medications contain aspirin or acetaminophen as well as caffeine and other drugs such as phenacetin, an effective aspirinlike analgesic that can harm the kidneys if taken in excessive amounts or over long periods of time. Some medications also contain salicylamide, an ingredient that studies have shown to be less effective than aspirin.

The caffeine present in combination remedies may help a headache by constricting blood vessels and acting as a mild stimulant. Too much caffeine, however, can cause nervousness and rapid heart rate and can even bring on a new headache. Also, these remedies almost always cost more than aspirin. Two plain aspirin or tablets of acetaminophen and a quarter cup of coffee may be a cheaper, safer way to get the same effect provided by OTC aspirin/caffeine combinations.

Over-the-counter drugs that claim to relieve sinus headaches often contain antihistamines. These antiallergy drugs may help allergy victims' headaches, but many sinus-headache sufferers have no allergies and therefore do not need antihistamines. Over-the-counter medications may also contain decongestants, but these drugs are often poorly absorbed when swallowed. In large doses, they may raise heart rate and blood pressure to dangerous levels.

In short, while some people obtain relief from OTC-combination headache remedies, many combinations are more expensive than aspirin, may carry more potential hazards, and are frequently not as effective.

INGREDIENTS OF SOME OTC COMBINATIONS

The composition of several popular brand-name pain relievers follows:

- Excedrin: 190 mg aspirin, 100 mg acetaminophen, 120 mg salicylamide, and 64 mg caffeine.

- Vanquish: 227 mg aspirin, 194 mg acetaminophen, 33 mg caffeine, and the antacids aluminum hydroxide and magnesium hydroxide.

- Anacin: 400 mg aspirin, 32 mg caffeine.

- Sinarest: 300 mg acetaminophen, 30 mg caffeine, 1 mg chlorpheniramine maleate (antihistamine), and 5 mg phenylephrine (decongestant).

- Sine-off: 325 mg aspirin, 2 mg chlorpheniramine maleate (antihistamine), 18.75 mg phenylpropanolamine (decongestant).

Another nonnarcotic pain reliever is ibuprofen, first available as the prescription drug Motrin but now sold without prescription as Nuprin or Advil. Ibuprofen was originally used to treat arthritis and severe menstrual cramps but has proved to be effective against headache. In general, it irritates the stomach less than aspirin does and is therefore recommended for people who cannot tolerate aspirin products. People allergic to aspirin, however, should not take ibuprofen without first consulting a physician because they may be similarly allergic to ibuprofen.

The narcotic analgesics doctors prescribe for headaches include codeine (sometimes stronger than aspirin); Percodan (a synthetic codeine); and meperidine (Demerol). Narcotics are often more effective against pain than nonprescription remedies and work by imitating the action of endorphins, the body's natural "stop pain" chemicals. Unfortunately, narcotic analgesics also have strong side effects, including nausea, vomiting, constipation, depression of breathing, loss of appetite, drowsiness, apathy, and even addiction. Moreover, because narcotics tend to become less effective over time against pain, the headache sufferer is forced to increase his or her dosages. For all these reasons, narcotics are not usually prescribed for ordinary headaches. For very severe head pain, however, they are sometimes given under a doctor's careful supervision.

Mood-altering drugs prescribed for headaches fall generally into two categories: tranquilizers (anxiety reducers) and antidepressants (mood elevators). Tranquilizers used against headaches include diazepam (Valium); chlordiazepoxide (Librium); meprobamate (Equanil); and phenobarbitol. As with the narcotic analgesics, these drugs are available only by prescription. Their side effects include drowsiness, loss of coordination, severe mood disturbances, and risk of addiction. Mood-altering drugs cannot relieve the pain of a headache that has already set in, but doctors sometimes prescribe them for people whose severe chronic headaches are set off by anxiety.

Antidepressants can help prevent headaches in two ways. First, if the sufferer is depressed, the medication will help him or her feel better in general. Second, some antidepressants help the body regulate its own pain-control mechanisms more efficiently. Antidepressants that prevent some severe chronic headaches include amitriptyline (Elavil) and imipramine (Tofranil).

Like tranquilizers, antidepressants have strong side effects: drowsiness, blurred vision, changes in heart rate and blood pressure, and numbness or tingling in the hands. In addition, people who take these drugs must strictly avoid certain foods such as chocolate, wine, nuts, aged cheeses, sour cream, and other foods that may cause a severe reaction when combined with antidepressant drugs. Like narcotic analgesics and tranquilizers, antidepressants are available only by prescription.

Special drugs that act directly against the physical causes of headaches include Parafon Forte, which is often prescribed for patients in whom muscle spasms or chronic muscle tension frequently trigger headaches. Other direct-action drugs for headache include ergotamine tartrate (Cafergot); methysergide (Sansert); and the heart medicine propranolol (Inderal). Because they have powerful and potentially dangerous side effects and because some may be habit-forming, special direct-action drugs are available only through a doctor's prescription, like other controlled drugs.

If you get a headache in spite of preventative measures, it is important to remember that all drugs—even the mildest—have side effects. Consequently, you may want to wait for the headache to go away by

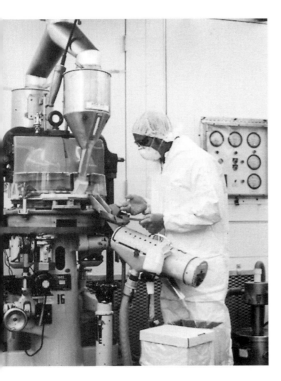

A chemist at a pharmaceutical company. Some of the more powerful drugs used to treat headaches have a number of serious side effects and are available by doctor's prescription only.

itself or try rest or meditation. If you are unable to shake your headache, however, and choose to take a pain reliever, use the mildest one—usually aspirin or acetaminophen—and take only the recommended dosage.

Most headaches are not dangerous in themselves, but a few may signal serious trouble. Thus, it is important to be alert to the headache signs and symptoms that call for medical attention.

5

DANGER-SIGNAL HEADACHES

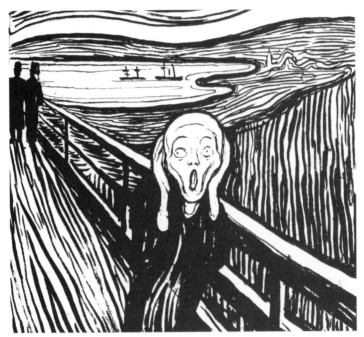

The Scream *by Edvard Munch.*

Most headaches are troublesome, painful—and innocent. Only a small percentage of head pain is caused by a brain tumor, a stroke, high blood pressure, or by any of the other serious illnesses people may worry about when they frequently suffer severe headaches. Only 1 in every 200–300 headaches suffered by an adult needs any treatment other than relief from pain.

There are rare headaches, however, that serve as warnings of serious illness and must be investigated promptly by a physician. The following guidelines can help you determine if a headache should be looked into.

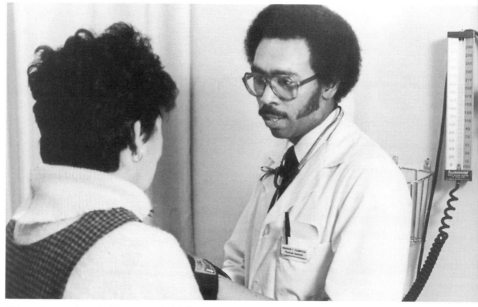

Although most headaches are painful, few are indications of a more serious problem. If the headache persists, however, and is accompanied by numbness, fever, or seizures, a physician should be consulted.

Sudden severe pain in any part of the body is one good reason to consult a physician. But pain alone does not indicate the seriousness of its cause. One person may have an agonizing headache that is not at all dangerous; another may have mild head pain that signals a life-threatening condition. Thus, the first question to ask oneself when deciding whether to consult a physician about a headache is, Does my headache represent a significant change in my health pattern?

A change in health pattern can mean several things. It may mean that someone used to getting only an occasional headache now suffers one almost every day. It may mean that the headache differs from previous headaches either in the intensity of the pain or in its location. Finally, a change in health pattern may consist of a health worry that just will not go away. No one wants to run to the doctor about every little question or anxiety, but someone with an ongoing concern about headaches should not hesitate to seek medical attention.

Specific headache symptoms that merit a visit to the doctor include the following:

- A sudden, very severe headache that seems to come out of nowhere, especially in someone who has never had such a headache before. Called a "thunderclap headache," this type of head pain may be a symptom of a leaking or burst blood vessel in the brain. Such an event may occur without warning in an apparently healthy person and is a potentially life-threatening emergency.

- A headache accompanied by uncontrollable twitching, numbness, weakness, or seizures—also called fits or convulsions. This may indicate a disorder of the brain or nervous system.

- A headache accompanied by a fever that has no obvious cause—in a person who does not have the flu or other illness, for instance. This may signal infection in the brain or spinal cord.

- A headache accompanied by confusion, loss of consciousness, irrational thinking or behavior, or any other change in normal mental state. This may come from a number of serious causes, including stroke, and deserves prompt attention and medical treatment.

- Headache along with pain in one spot, such as the eye, ear, or neck—especially a stiff neck. This can be a warning signal of infection or other serious illness.

- Recurring headaches in children. These should always be treated as warning signs because children's headaches represent serious illness more often than adult headaches do. Any sudden change in a child's headache, even when the child has a clear cause for the headache, such as the flu, demands investigation because it can mean the start of a brain infection.

- Recurring headaches that begin suddenly in a person who has not had them before. These should be investigated because they represent a dangerous change in the person's health pattern.

- Headaches that worsen when the victim coughs, stoops, or strains—when lifting a heavy object, for example. This may signal high blood pressure, blockage in the brain, or other serious illness. Similarly, headaches that awaken a person at night or that interfere with daily activities should be reported to a physician as well.

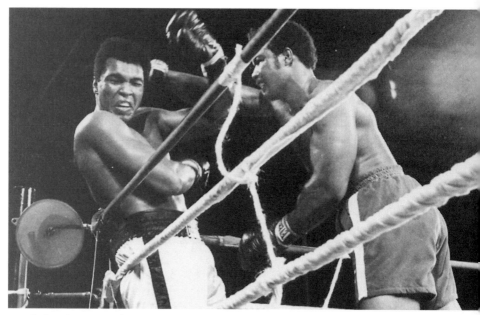

Headaches that occur after a head injury, such as one sustained during a boxing match, should be checked by a physician as soon as possible. Such injuries can result in skull fracture or brain damage.

- Headaches that occur frequently in elderly persons—especially in women over the age of 60. These need prompt attention by a doctor because they may signal a disease of blood vessels in the head, temporal arteritis, that can cause blindness if not treated.

- Headaches occurring after head injury. These need treatment because head injury is the cause of death in two-thirds of people who die under the age of 35. Falls, auto accidents, and sports mishaps can cause head injuries that result in skull fracture or brain damage.

  A blow to the head can injure the brain in two ways. In the *coup* injury, the brain is damaged at the spot where the head is struck; in the *contrecoup* injury, the spot farthest from the blow is damaged when the force of the blow pushes or pulls the brain against or away from the skull, literally making the brain bounce inside the head.

The key question after head injury is whether or not the injury is minor (uncomplicated concussion) or major. In major head injury, internal bleeding occurs and rapidly increases pressure in the skull and damages the brain, often permanently, sometimes fatally. In a minor head injury, no such bleeding occurs.

The victim of uncomplicated concussion may be unconscious—"out cold"—for a few seconds immediately after the blow to the head. Upon coming to, the victim has a visual disturbance: he or she "sees stars." Dizziness, a headache, and amnesia—forgetting what happened in the moments before the mishap—are also concussion symptoms. Anyone who suffers a concussion should see a physician as soon as possible in order to rule out brain damage, the signs of which may not be obvious. If the victim does not regain consciousness at once after a blow to the head, his or her life may be in danger, and emergency medical help should be summoned at once.

If a person wakes up immediately after a head injury but becomes unconscious again later, or if drowsiness, irrational speech, vomiting, severe headache, or any other abnormal behavior occurs, the victim

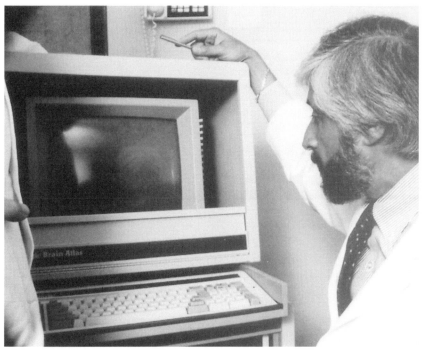

A doctor studies a computer assessment of a head injury, which is the cause of death in two-thirds of people who die under the age of 35.

should be taken to a physician or hospital emergency room at once because these symptoms may signal rapidly developing brain damage.

If a person suffers no obvious ill effects from a blow to the head but begins having chronic or severe headaches soon afterward, he or she should be examined by a physician, who can determine the reason for the headaches, rule out serious causes, and possibly cure the ailment.

Again, most headaches are not serious, but a few do warn of potentially serious conditions. Young people or their family members who have any of the warning-sign headaches should see a doctor as soon as possible, just to be on the safe side. The doctor may treat the headache—or just ease the worry—but either way, medical attention is definitely called for with a danger-sign headache.

6

MIGRAINE: THE ONE-SIDED PAIN

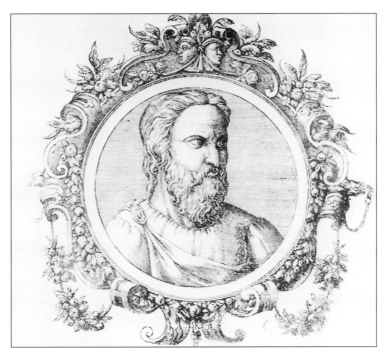

Aretaeus

n A.D. 100, the Alexandrian physician Aretaeus had this to say about migraine headaches:

> In certain cases the whole head is pained, and the pain is sometimes on the right and sometimes on the left side, or the forehead, and attacks may shift their place during the same day. The illness includes nausea, vomiting, collapse . . . heaviness of the head, anxiety, and life becomes a burden. [Victims] flee the light; darkness soothes their disease. . . . They are weary of life and wish to die.

Today's migraine sufferers—approximately 6% of men and 18% of women in the United States alone—will readily recognize Aretaeus's account. It describes many familiar symptoms and also captures the mercurial nature of migraines. From victim to victim, from one attack to the next, and even within a single attack, pain and other unpleasant symptoms of migraine may change their type, their intensity, and their location.

The frequency with which migraine attacks occur also varies widely. In 1960, Dr. J. W. Lance of the University of Sydney, in Australia, studied 500 patients. He found that 15% suffered more than 10 attacks per month and that about half suffered between 1 and 4 attacks per month. Lance reported these results in the *Journal of Neurology and Neurosurgery*. In 1966, Lance repeated his study and arrived at the same results, which he reported in *Archives of Neurology*. Some migraines run in cycles, occurring several times a week for a period of weeks and then vanishing entirely until the next cycle begins. A few unfortunate sufferers have migraine headaches every day.

Yet another point of variance is the underlying causes of migraines. In some cases the headache may be brought on by strong emotion; in others, a bite of cheese or sip of wine can trigger it. Stimulation of senses may cause pain in migraine-prone persons; some can bring on an attack by sniffing an unpleasant odor or staring at patterned wallpaper, others simply by considering such mild actions.

The exact physical cause of migraine eludes medical science. No structural abnormality has been clearly identified in the brains of victims. Moreover, the sufferer often feels perfectly healthy between attacks except for the knowledge that another migraine is sure to strike again sooner or later. This, in fact, is one of the few reliable features of migraine: it almost always comes back.

The best-known migraine symptom is the pain itself. In two-thirds of the victims of *common migraine,* the headache comes on as a violent throbbing in one temple (the side of the head near the forehead); in the rest, the pain occurs on both sides of the head from the start of the attack. The throbbing may subside into a steady intense ache that can last from a few minutes to as long as a week or more. The headache is often accompanied by photophobia—extreme sensitivity to light.

The other usual feature of common migraine is nausea. Sometimes it is mild; other times it can be so severe that even the idea of food causes vomiting. In addition, the sufferer may feel general misery, a disgust not only with food but also with everything. In this state, almost any environment makes the victim feel worse, except darkness and silence.

About one-third of migraine victims have a form of the ailment called *classical migraine,* wherein the headache, nausea, and light sensitivity are accompanied by varying symptoms of nervous-system disorder. Sufferers of classical migraine—so called because it is the kind often mentioned in famous victims' writings—include Julius Caesar, Saint Paul, philosopher Immanuel Kant and the father of psychoanalysis, Sigmund Freud.

Together, classical migraine's nervous-system symptoms are known as the aura, or disturbance in one or more of the physical senses. When these symptoms affect sight, as they do in about one-third of classical migraine sufferers, they may manifest as blurred or shimmering vision, flashing light, or colors that zigzag across the field of vision.

Some migraine victims see strange, complex visual auras; these may trouble children, who may mistake these visions for actual threats and who may be afraid to talk about them for fear of being disbelieved or punished. Migrainous sight disturbances may also cause temporary spots of blindness called *scotoma* (the Latin word for "shadow of darkness").

One possible explanation for visual migraine auras has been discovered by Harvard scientist and migraine victim Dr. K. S. Lashley. As the visual auras of his migraine came on, he measured the decrease in his vision by marking the edges of his blind-spot with lines of stickpins pushed into a screen he kept staring at. Using his blind-spot map, Dr. Lashley later calculated that the cortex of his brain (the part where sight is processed) was being affected by a process—whose exact operation was unknown to him—that moved at a rate of three millimeters per minute.

In fact there is a known process that moves across the cortex at just the rate Dr. Lashley calculated. It is called spreading depression and is accompanied first by the constriction of blood vessels and then by their dilation—the same blood-vessel disturbances thought to play a large role in migraine pain.

Other experiments have shown that when the cortex is affected by a spreading depression, a person sees zigzag patterns; when the cortex is affected all at once, he or she sees stars. Other migraine auras include tingling or numbness of the hands, tongue, or mouth; hearing illusory sounds so vivid the victim thinks a radio is playing; imaginary odors— often strong and repulsive—and other sense upsets. These auras may be caused by changes in the nerve cells of the brain, but no one has yet even gathered all the pieces of the migraine puzzle together, much less

YOUNG HEADACHE VICTIMS

The pictures shown on these two pages were drawn by young headache sufferers treated at the Michigan Headache and Neurological Institute. The first drawing in each pair was done by a child before he or she received treatment, the second after the child had recovered.

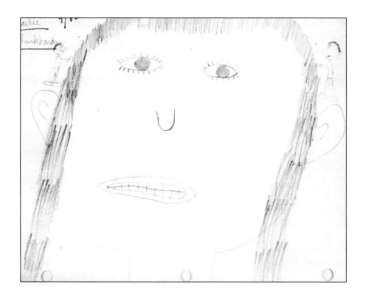

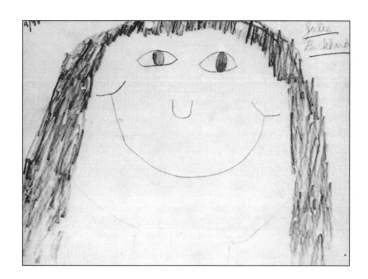

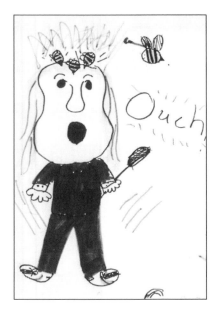

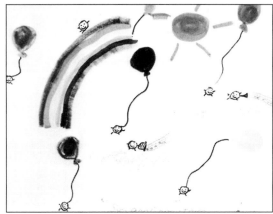

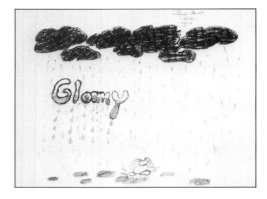

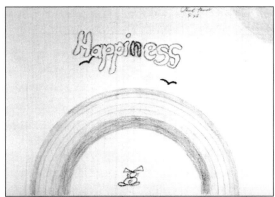

assembled them into a complete picture of just how and why migraine and its auras occur.

Another common, intense aura symptom is *vertigo* (dizziness), which can be so severe that the victim cannot walk until the attack passes. A migraine aura may also prevent the victim from speaking, writing, or thinking with normal clarity. Emotions, too, may be affected: the victim may feel amused, guilty, frightened, or simply strange—all the while knowing that there is no external reason for the feelings.

Whatever their specific nature, migraine auras have these elements in common: they occur suddenly and last for a short time; they have no physical basis aside from the migraine itself; they feel overwhelmingly real to the sufferer; they are accompanied by a sense of "time standing still"; finally, the victim finds the sensation of the aura defies explanation.

Classical migraine auras often occur before the onset of headache and last for 20 to 45 minutes. Common and classical migraine victims learn to note other warning signs as well. One such is a mood change—feeling unusually wonderful and energetic, for instance, or drowsy with frequent yawning. Another is a dramatic change in appetite and cravings for certain foods—often for chocolate or other sweets.

Just as the symptoms of migraine vary, so do its sufferers. Migraine victims range from young children to the elderly and include artists, teachers, and truck drivers; 60%–75%, however, have relatives who also get migraines. Thus, it is believed that a tendency to develop the ailment is inherited.

Indeed, experts think that the child of a migraine sufferer has more than a 50% chance of inheriting the affliction, often before the age of 15. A survey reported in the Danish medical journal *Clinical Aspects of Migraine* showed that only about 3% of 7 year olds and 9% of 15 year olds have migraines. By age 19, however, the number rises to about 19% in women, with about 11% of 19-year-old men suffering from migraines.

Not all these young people will continue to have headaches throughout their life, but 60% will be plagued into adulthood. Some may appear to "outgrow" the ailment during their young-adult years only to have it reappear later in life. Still other sufferers lose the pain but not the aura; they retain sight disturbances and other nervous-system symptoms, a condition known as migraine equivalent. Finally, people who begin having migraines as adults, or who continue to have attacks that began in youth, may find that as they grow older they suffer fewer or less frequent headaches. Seventy percent of such adults report that headaches diminish in severity and frequency as they grow older. An interesting fact is that women get migraines more often than men, by a ratio of about 3 to 1.

TREATMENT FOR MIGRAINE HEADACHES

Because the causes and symptoms of migraine are various and complex, treatment of the disorder is complicated, too. In his book *Migraine,* Dr. Oliver Sacks explains the diversity of treatment methods available. "Some patients I help with drugs, and some with the magic of attention and interest. Some defeated my therapeutic maneuvers until I started to inquire minutely . . . into their emotional lives."

Migraine is so complicated, Sacks suggests, because it is not only a biologic event but an emotional and intellectual one as well. It is, as he puts it, a "prototype of a psychophysiological reaction."

In short, a migraine headache is often not just a physical pain, or just an emotional pain, or just a pain of the mind. It may be all these things,

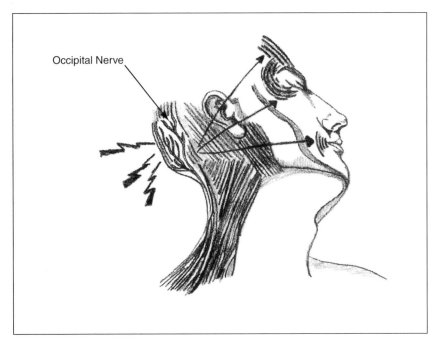

Figure 5: The Path of Migraine Pain.

all at the same time. No wonder, then, that migraine has confused doctors and victims alike throughout history.

Nevertheless, progress has been made in the search for causes, prevention, and treatment of migraine headaches. Many doctors believe the pain of migraine occurs when a blood vessel in the head suddenly constricts and then just as suddenly dilates.

But what starts the cycle of squeeze, stretch, and pain in the first place? Researchers now believe that brain activity starts the cycle. One theory suggests that a wave of lowered nervous-system activity runs along the nerves in the brain's surface, lowering the level of oxygen there and triggering blood vessel spasms that result in pain. A study conducted by James Dexter, a researcher at the University of Missouri and president of the American Association for the Study of Headaches, measured the brain-wave activity in migraine victims and found that half the subjects experienced a slowing of brain waves during attacks.

It is not yet clear what triggers the slowdown, but it seems that if a person has inherited sensitive brain-wave slowing mechanisms, they may be triggered by many causes—different foods, sights, sounds, and other irritants. A single brain "trigger" may be pulled by many "fingers." One such inherited trigger may be an excess or deficiency in brain chemicals. These chemicals, including norepinephrine, serotonin, and prostaglandin, belong to the body's pain transmission system and help regulate the way pain impulses are sent.

Chemicals that are eaten or drunk may be trigger-pulling fingers that affect the way the body's pain chemicals are produced or distributed. Foods such as bacon, chocolate, Chinese food, and alcohol are among the many items that cause migraine headaches in those sensitive to them. These food items contain chemicals such as tyramine, nitrates, caffeine, and monosodium glutamate, whose precise effects on the brain chemistry are not entirely known.

Some women get migraine headaches only during their menstrual periods, when their level of progesterone, a hormone, falls. Once such women become pregnant and their progesterone levels rise, their headaches vanish until their child is born—and then the headaches return. The exact action of progesterone on headache-pain causes is not yet fully understood.

Stress, a well-known migraine-headache cause, may also produce changes in brain chemicals or affect the pain-control system in other,

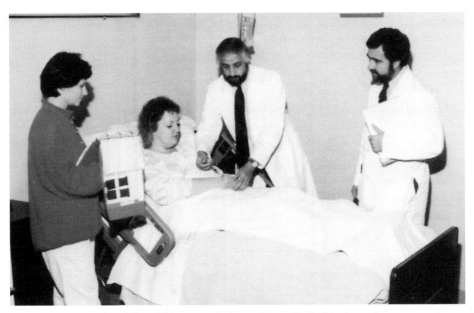

Dr. Alvin Lake of the Michigan Headache and Neurological Institute observes a patient undergoing biofeedback, a method that enables patients to control the flow of blood in their bodies.

unknown ways. In general, stress is emotional pressure. A student worried about an upcoming exam, for example, may feel a great deal of conflicting pressures. Parents and teachers may urge the student to prepare diligently and do well, whereas friends may encourage him or her to go out or attend a special event. The result may be stress—and a migraine headache.

Stress-caused migraines are apt to strike once the cause of the stress has ended—when the victim relaxes. This reinforces scientists' theory that vessel widening after the anxiety-caused constriction is a cause of migraine, but it is probably not the whole answer.

Still, stress control—learning how to cope with pressure—is one of the main ways doctors are helping migraine victims to prevent headache. Avoiding known causes of migraine—foods, drinks, situations, and activities that a sufferer knows will bring on an attack—helps prevent migraines, too.

Some people have learned to regulate blood flow in their own brain and thus reduce migraine pain by a method called biofeedback; to become effective, this method of controlling migraine requires special training with scientific instruments. Once a person knows how to do it, however, no machinery is needed. Biofeedback and other headache treatments will be discussed more fully in Chapter 8.

Drugs Used to Treat Migraines

Drugs useful in treating migraine fall into two categories, those that prevent attacks and those useful in stopping attacks that have already begun. Preventives include antidepressants such as Elavil, which alters pain chemicals in the brain; drugs such as Inderal and calcium channel blockers, which treat spasms of blood vessels; and antiinflammatories such as ibuprofen, which acts on blood vessels and block some pain impulses.

There are drugs that treat migraines that have already begun. One that is effective against severe pain is a synthetic version of ergot, a fungus that grows on grain, especially rye. Ergot was first found to work against headaches more than 60 years ago. Ergotamine is given in various forms: by injection, inhalation, suppository, or placed under the tongue for absorption. Ergotamine works by constricting swollen pain-producing blood vessels, but it can cause headaches itself and so is only given until the victim is well enough to try other, less drastic treatments. Another drug, sumatriptan (Imitrex), works by increasing the effects of serotonin in the body. Low levels of serotonin may cause migraines. Sumatriptan may be taken orally or by injection.

Migraine headaches rarely pose any danger, but they can seriously disrupt the life of those who suffer them. Thus, these headaches should be treated by a physician, for while there is still no cure, modern medicine can lessen their pain and can sometimes even banish them for good.

7

BIG-TIME HELP FOR BIG-TIME HEADACHES

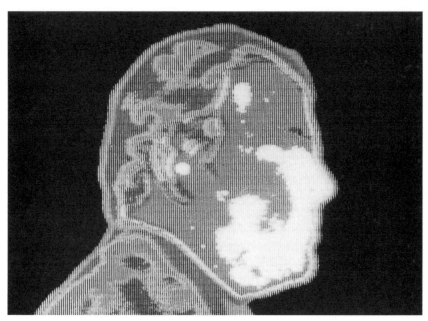

Thermography

Because most people do not get terrible headaches, life is harder for the few who do. They must endure not only pain, nausea, and other symptoms of their special misery but also the misunderstanding of those around them.

Relatives and friends of chronic headache sufferers may think that the victim is making a big deal of a little discomfort. Families who must repeatedly cancel plans on account of one family member's headache may lose sympathy as the disappointments pile up. If no specific medical cause for the headaches can be found, even the victim's family doctor may make statements such as "You'll just have to learn to live with it" and "You've got to try to relax."

On top of their pain, headache victims suffer anxiety, loneliness, helplessness, and guilt. They have nowhere to turn and begin to suspect their friends and relatives may be right. Perhaps, the sufferer thinks, I am at fault for my headache. Since the late 1970s, however, doctors have started to recognize that chronic severe headaches are a real and destructive problem. Thus, a few full-time headache clinics have sprung up throughout the United States. At these places, physicians identify and treat chronic headache as a disease in its own right, one that can be diagnosed, prevented, and treated, if not cured. Victims benefit from the work of a team approach to investigation and treatment that involves doctors, nurses, psychologists, psychiatrists, and other professionals.

Some patients are sent to headache clinics by their family doctors; some enter the clinics of their own accord. (Names and addresses of headache clinics and other information sources appear in the Appendix to this book.) No matter what leads them to a headache clinic, most patients find sympathy, understanding, and assistance—often for the first time in their life.

When a patient first visits a clinic the specialists there review a history of the patient's headaches. This information enables the staff to determine adequate treatment from the outset. Commonly, three separate clinic appointments, each lasting as long as an hour or more, are needed for the team to collect all the necessary information.

In the first information-gathering step, a complete physical examination is performed on the patient (if any blood tests or X rays are required, they are administered), and a staff member takes a detailed medical and surgical history of the patient and reviews the history of his or her family in order to determine if any close relatives have headache problems. Most important, the patient discusses every detail of his or her headache, both in a questionnaire and in an interview with a doctor or other member of the clinic staff.

Patients are asked how the headaches feel, how often they occur, and what part of the head is affected. They are then encouraged to describe what they think brings on the headaches—particular foods, activities, situations, mood changes, emotions, and so on. They explain the treatments they have tried in the past and whether or not any of these methods have helped. Patients also list the medications they are presently taking or have taken.

The patient also tells the clinic staff about his or her personality and attitudes and about specific stresses he or she faces in daily life. A psychologist may also give the patient a personality test. The patient answers questions about how the headaches affect him or her and how life would change if the headaches went away. All this information allows the clinic staff to treat the patient as a unique person rather than as "just another headache."

During the second visit to the clinic, laboratory tests are often conducted to determine how the patient's body is behaving during headaches and in between. The patient's muscle tension is charted painlessly with a special device called an electromyograph. The test is administered in the following fashion. First, sensors are taped to the skin to measure muscle reactions. Next, a technician asks the patient certain questions and invites him or her to imagine different activities and to think about various situations. Meanwhile, the patient's changing muscle activity is recorded on an electromyogram. The technician also records such information as the temperature of the patient's hands.

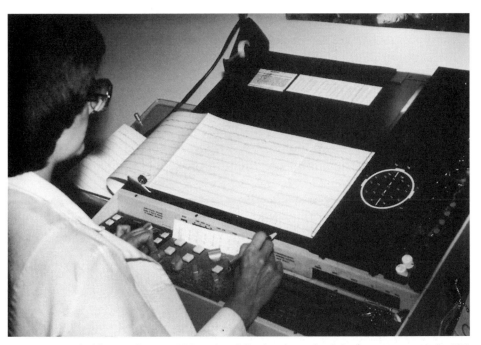

A technician conducts an EEG tracing, following the patient's brain-wave pattern. An EEG can be used to determine if a patient has epilepsy or simply to check on how well the nerves in the head function.

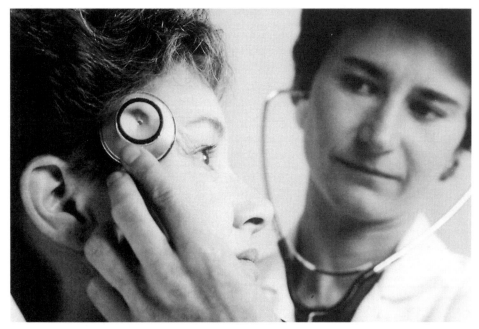

In a test called a Doppler study, the physician listens through earphones to the blood flow in the patient's head.

Information gathered from these tests can provide important clues about the causes of the headaches. The temperature of the hands, for instance, is a measure of blood flow; cold hands suggest the patient may have migraine headaches. Strong muscle contractions may signal that the patient suffers tension headaches. Some patients have cold hands *and* tense muscles; they may have a combination of tension and migraine headaches.

Other tests done at the clinic measure the proper functioning of the nervous system. An electroencephalogram (EEG), for example, shows the brain-wave pattern. Technicians tape sensors to the patient's head to measure electrical activity in the brain to determine if the patient has an underlying disease such as epilepsy, a disorder at the central nervous system marked by disturbed electrical rhythms and causing convulsions. Other examinations performed by the doctor test how well the nerves in the head work.

Often the doctor will also listen through earphones to the blood flow in the head, in a test called the Doppler study. In another test, a thermogram, a special photograph taken of the patient's face can indicate the possible presence of painfully widened arteries. The patient's vision, hearing, coordination, and reflexes are also examined for abnormalities in these areas or in the nerves controlling them.

Yet another exam, a computerized axial tomography (CAT) scan, checks for a tumor, blood clot, or other abnormality in the patient's brain by means of an X ray that photographs the inside of the patient's head and allows physicians to inspect tiny areas deep inside the brain. Because CAT scanners are so costly, the test is usually available only in a hospital. However, it is almost always done on an outpatient basis; that is, the patient goes to the hospital to have the test done but leaves shortly thereafter. Like the tests done at the clinic, a CAT scan is painless.

Once all the tests and examinations have been done and the results evaluated, the clinic doctor meets with the patient once again to

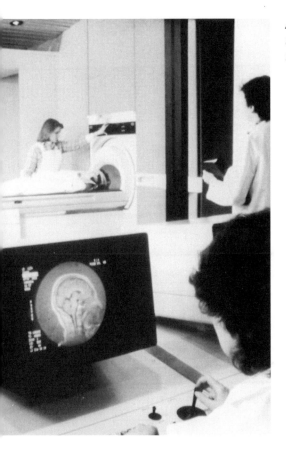

A CAT scanner, shown here, checks for tumor, blood clot, and other abnormalities in the patient's brain.

explain what has been learned. The doctor outlines an individualized treatment plan, the goal of which is to lessen headache frequency, severity, and duration if it seems the ailment cannot be banished altogether. In general, the plan aims to eliminate the need for narcotic painkillers and to reduce use of OTC analgesics as much as possible. The specifics of the plan differ for almost every patient, though it often includes changes in diet, such as smaller, more frequent meals and avoidance of certain foods, and in behavior, such as more or less sleep and new exercise habits.

Patients often receive psychological therapy to help emotional and stress difficulties. Some receive relaxation therapy that teaches them to relieve muscle-tension habits that bring on headaches. Some learn biofeedback, a method for controlling automatic body functions such as blood flow to painful areas in the head. (Biofeedback and relaxation therapy are described in more detail in Chapter 8.) For most patients, the treatment plan contains some elements of all these therapies. If necessary, the doctor prescribes medication.

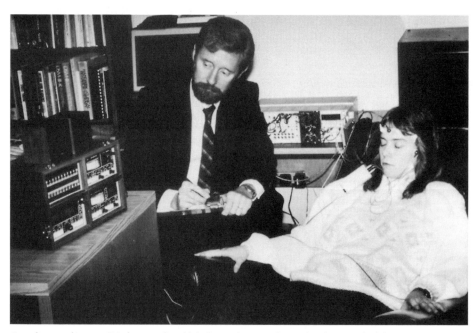

A patient undergoes I.V. therapy, in which the patient receives migraine-treating drugs intravenously.

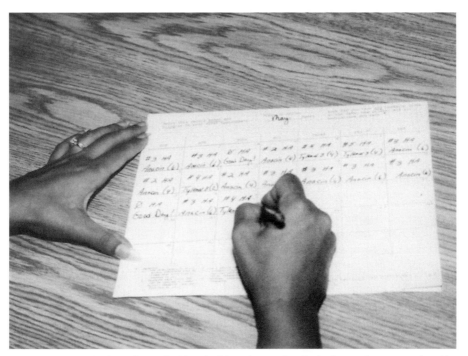

Some headache sufferers find it valuable to keep a headache log and may even be able to detect a pattern after a period of time.

Besides following the treatment plan and taking medicines, a headache-clinic patient keeps a journal to record the frequency, severity, and length of his or her headaches. Patients also keep a record of the medicines they take and list other information, such as what they were doing and what they had eaten when a headache occurred. Each time the patient visits the clinic for a follow-up visit, the physician consults the journal to see how well the treatment has been working for the patient. In this way the doctor can tell whether or not the plan needs to be changed.

At the outset of the treatment, or if the patient's headaches prove unusually difficult to control, the doctor may schedule follow-up visits. Gradually, the patient visits the clinic less often, although he or she can call an emergency number in the event a sudden, severe headache strikes when the clinic is not open. In that case, the doctor often meets the patient at a local hospital emergency room and promptly provides evaluation and care.

The treatment given at a headache clinic demands considerable effort on the part of the patient, who must answer questions, undergo tests, follow the treatment plan, keep careful records, and show up regularly for additional appointments. Moreover, clinics are expensive: The cost of initial visits plus laboratory and other tests can total over $1,000 (a portion of which may be covered by the patient's health insurance).

Nonetheless, headache clinics treat children, young people, and adults with success; 90% of the time, the patient either improves dramatically or recovers completely.

8

A PAIN-FREE TOMORROW?

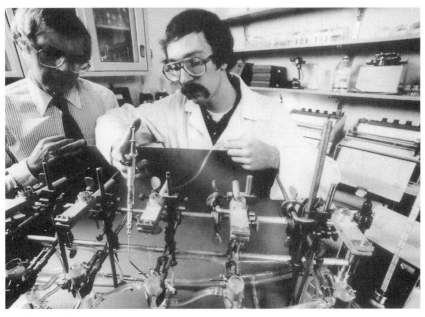

Testing new drugs.

Progress is being made against headaches, but scientific research into their causes and cures is difficult because the ailment afflicts an area of the body that remains, to some extent, a mystery. Medical researchers still lack conclusive answers to questions about the brain (what it is and how it works) and about the nervous system (the path by which pain impulses travel). And because emotions play a big part in headaches—in their origins, the intensity of the pain, and in our reactions to that pain—knowledge about headaches requires a study of how emotions are caused, controlled, and felt.

The investigation of the physical nature of headache is complicated further because, as was mentioned earlier, animals evidently do not suffer headaches and thus cannot be used in laboratory experiments. In fact, until recently, almost all that was known about headaches was what headache sufferers reported.

Yet another obstacle to headache research is the scarcity of funds available to subsidize it. Drs. Walter Stewart of Johns Hopkins University and Martha Linet of the National Cancer Institute had to apply three times to the National Institutes of Health (NIH) for a small grant to fund a survey of young-adult headache sufferers. The problem was not that the NIH faulted the survey but that the organization spends only about $1 million per year on headache studies. By contrast, the annual outlay for heart disease research is over $600 million. The money that is available for headache research comes from two main sources: private investors—drug companies hoping to find a new headache cure they can sell, for instance—and public tax money. Both sources saddle researchers with strict budgets.

Despite such obstacles, scientists have made major strides toward finding causes of and cures for headaches. For instance, researcher Dr. John Meyer studied blood flow in the head during migraine attacks, using a special helmet that shows changes in circulation. His work confirms the idea that blood vessels inside the head do contract and then expand during migraine attacks.

Studies of chemicals in the body are also giving scientists new answers. The blood level of serotonin, for instance, drops in migraine but remains constant in cluster headaches, while the level of blood histamine rises sharply in cluster headaches but only a bit in migraine. Just what these results mean is not yet clear, but what is clear is that in some way migraine differs physically from cluster headaches.

NEW TREATMENT OPTIONS

Some specialists find new nondrug techniques offer effective treatment. These techniques allow the headache sufferer to feel that he or she has some control over his or her own pain. At the same time, these techniques have few or none of the side effects created by most drug therapies. Some of these nondrug therapies include the following.

Biofeedback Biofeedback is a method for learning to voluntarily regulate body functions not ordinarily under a person's conscious control, such as blood pressure, heart rate, or digestion. In biofeedback, the body's functions are monitored by an electronic device that translates the body's activities into signals such as clicking sounds or flashing lights. The technique is so potent that by training on an electroencephalograph (EEG)—a machine that measures brain waves and displays a graph of the waves on paper or on a screen machine—some people have even learned to control their own brain waves.

To help a person control migraine headaches, feedback sensors are first taped to the hand. As blood flow to the hand rises and falls, clicking sounds made by the device speed up and slow down. The patient uses these signals as a guide and can gradually learn to control blood flow in the hand and also to direct blood flow to or away from it. He or she then learns to do the same thing for the head, sending blood flow away from the pain and thereby vanquishing it. A person trained and practiced in the technique may perform it without conscious thought.

Relaxation Therapy   Aimed at lessening physical and mental stress, relaxation therapy is sometimes used in conjunction with biofeedback. A main point taught by relaxation therapists is that relaxing is not a passive but a conscious process. Simply ceasing strenuous activity is not enough; someone can be tense even while lying on a sofa.

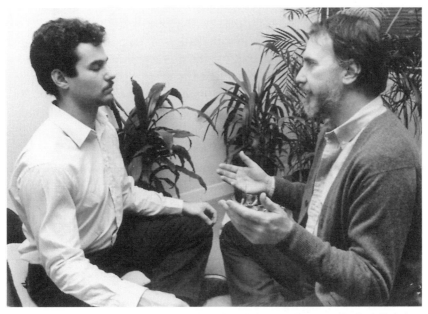

Relaxation therapy involves learning how to relax all the muscles in the body deliberately. This method is particularly effective for a patient suffering from a tension headache.

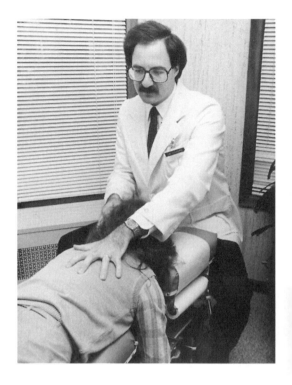

A chiropractor checks a patient. Chiropractors believe that some pain may be caused by a subluxation of the bones in the neck, which in turn press on the nerves radiating from the spinal cord.

There are many methods for learning how to relax; most include such exercises as spending a period of time in a quiet place, focusing all one's attention on a single object, sound, or thought, and sitting or lying in a comfortable position. Once the patient has done this, he or she can proceed to think deliberately about the muscles and then relax them, one by one, starting with the toes, going on to the feet, the ankles, the lower legs, and so on, until all the muscles are as relaxed as possible.

Once a tension headache victim masters relaxation exercises, he or she does them every day, whether or not a headache is present. This prevents muscle-tension habits from returning—and can help lessen the frequency and intensity of tension headaches.

TENS   Transcutaneous electrical nerve stimulation (TENS) uses tiny doses of electricity to block pain signals to the brain. TENS is safe, has no known side effects, and is believed effective in the treatment of some forms of chronic pain. However, many headache experts consider its use experimental and are not sure it really works against headaches.

Chiropractic Treatment   Chiropractors believe some pain and diseases are caused by a subluxation (incorrect or abnormal position) of the bones in the neck, which press on nerves that radiate from the spinal cord and can be manipulated into alignment by a trained practitioner.

Acupuncture   In the United States, acupuncture—an ancient Chinese medical therapy—has proved a controversial method of treating and preventing headaches. Acupuncture consists of the insertion of needles into areas of the skin prescribed by ancient Chinese medical teachings. Some people say acupuncture helps; others say it amounts to a placebo, meaning it works because the patient believes in its effectiveness.

But this skepticism is colored by cultural differences. In China, acupuncture works so well as a painkiller that it is used as an anesthetic during major surgery. The patient who tries acupuncture should be careful, however. Diseases such as hepatitis (a liver disease) and acquired immune deficiency syndrome ([AIDS], a fatal disease that causes the

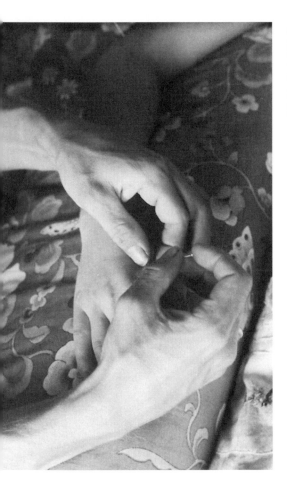

Acupuncture is a controversial method of treatment for headache sufferers. Those who are opposed to this method believe that people only feel it is working because they expect it to—the placebo effect.

breakdown of the body's immune system) may be spread by dirty needles. Thus, patients must make sure their practitioner is qualified and uses sterilized needles.

WHAT CAN BE DONE, WHAT WILL BE ACCOMPLISHED?

Until medical science finds the ultimate headache cure, healthful living, stress control, and relaxation will continue to be the keys to preventing common headaches, and mild analgesics such as aspirin will remain the preferred treatment. For more severe headaches, a doctor's office is the best place to find relief.

By the time today's young people are raising their own families, more help may be available to combat all kinds of headaches. In the meantime, headache sufferers and their families can take heart from this fact: new and growing medical knowledge about headache causes, preventions, and cures offers better relief from headaches than at any previous time in human history, and the prospect for the future improves each day.

APPENDIX

FOR MORE INFORMATION

Below are the names and addresses of national organizations that can provide further information on headaches.

American Council for
    Headache Education
875 Kings Highway, Suite 200
Woodbury, NJ 08096
www.achenet.org

American Headache Society
19 Mantua Rd.
Mt. Royal, NJ 08061
(856) 423-0043
www.aash.org

National Institute of Neurological
    Disorders and Stroke
National Institute of Health
Bethesda, MD 20892
www.ninds.nih.gov

National Headache Foundation
5252 N. Western Avenue
Chicago, IL 60625
(312) 878-7715
www.headaches.org

The following is a sampling of clinics around the country that can provide information and treatment for headaches.

Headache Treatment Center
Cedars Medical Center, Inc.
1295 NW 14th St.
Miami, FL 33125
(305) 325-4520

Headache Treatment Center
Georgetown University Medical Center
3800 Reservoir Rd.
Washington, DC 20007
(202) 625-0100

Houston Headache Clinic
1213 Hermann Dr. #350
Houston, TX 77004
(713) 528-1916

Michigan Headache and
    Neurological Institute
3120 Professional Drive
Ann Arbor, MI 48104
(734) 677-6000
www.mhni.com

Minnesota Headache Institute
5851 Duluth St., Suite 204
Minneapolis, MN 55422
(612) 588-0661

Mt. Sinai Headache Clinic
1031 Fifth Ave.
New York, NY 10028
(212) 650-7691

San Francisco Headache Clinic
909 Hyde St., Suite 230
San Francisco, CA 92109
(415) 673-4600
www.citilinks.com/headache/sfhcjc.htm

University of Missouri
Department of Neurology
Columbia, MO 65212
(573) 884-4249
www.muhealth.org/~brain/

University of New Mexico
Department of Neurology
915 Camino de Salud NE
Albuquerque, NM 87131
(505) 272-3342
salud.unm.edu/neuro/

APPENDIX

FURTHER READING

Antonovosky, Aaron. *Unraveling the Mystery of Health: How People Manage Stress and Stay Well.* San Francisco: Jossey-Bass, 1987.

Appley, Mortimer H., and Richard Trumbell, eds. *Dynamics of Stress: Physiological, Psychological, and Social Perspectives.* New York: Plenum, 1986.

Benson, Herbert, M.D. *The Relaxation Response.* New York: Avon Books 1975.

Clark, M. "Headaches." *Newsweek* 110 (December 7, 1987): 76–82.

Constantine, Lynn M. *Migraine: The Complete Guide.* New York: Dell, 1994.

Dalsgarrd-Neilsen, T. "Some Aspects of the Epidemiology of Migraine." *Clinical Aspects of Migraine.* Nordlundes Bogtrykker, 1970.

Diamond, Seymour, M.D., and William Barry Furlong. *More Than Two Aspirin: Hope for Your Headache Problem.* New York: Avon Books, 1976.

Dobson, C. B. *Stress, the Hidden Adversary.* Ridgewood, NJ: G. A. Bogden, 1983.

Elkind, Arthur. Migraines: *Everything You Need to Know About Their Cause and Cure.* New York: Avon, 1997.

Freese, Arthur S., D.D.S. *Headaches: The Kinds and the Cures.* Garden City, NY: Doubleday, 1973.

Krabbe, A. A., and J. Oleson. "Headaches Provocation by Continuous Infusion of Histamines." *Pain* 8 (1980): 253.

Lance, James W., M.D. *Migraine and Other Headaches.* New York: Scribner, 1986.

———, et al. "Treatment of Chronic Tension Headache." *Lancet* 1 (June 1963): 1236–39.

———, and G. Selby. "Observations on 500 Cases of Migraine." *The Journal of Neurology, Neurosurgery, and Psychiatry* 23 (1960): 23.

———, and M. Anthony. "Some Clinical Aspects of Migraine." *Archives of Neurosurgery* 15 (1966): 356.

Peterson, Christina, and Christine Adamec, *The Women's Migraine Survival Guide.* New York: Harper, 1999.

Physicians' Desk Reference for Nonprescription Drugs. Montvale, NJ: Medical Economics, 1999.

Rapoport, Alan M., M.D., Fred D. Sheftell, M.D., and Lucy Labson. "Health and Medical Horizons." In *Headaches.* New York: Macmillan, 1984.

————, R. Allan Purdy, and Fred D. Sheftell. *Advanced Therapy of Headache.* Phila.: BC Deker, 1998.

Rodgers, Joann Ellison. *Drugs and Pain.* New York: Chelsea House, 1987.

Sacks, Oliver. *Migraine.* Revised and expanded edition. New York: Vintage, 1999.

Saper, Joel R., M.D., and Kenneth R. Magee, M.D. *Freedom from Headaches.* New York: Simon & Schuster, 1986.

Scarry, Elaine. *The Body in Pain: The Making and Unmaking of the World.* New York: Oxford University Press, 1985.

Sicuteri, F. "Vasalactive Substances and Their Implications in Vascular Pain." Vol. 1, *Research and Clinical Studies in Headache.* New York and Basel: Karger, 1967.

Spierings, Egiluis. *Headache.* Stoneham, MA: Butterworth, 1998.

Zimmerman, David R. *The Essential Guide to Nonprescription Drugs.* New York: Harper & Row, 1983.

APPENDIX

GLOSSARY

Acetaldehyde: A toxic by-product of alcohol digestion.

Acetaminophen: A white, odorless crystalline powder; used as an analgesic and antifever medication; brand names include Tylenol.

Acetate: A toxic by-product of alcohol digestion.

Acetylcholine: A neurotransmitter that is thought to play an important role in transmitting impulses along nerves.

Acetylsalicylic acid: The synthetic form of salicylic acid; the active ingredient in aspirin.

Acupuncture: Ancient Chinese method of pain relief, performed by inserting needles under the skin at prescribed points that correspond to various internal organs and functions; particular point to cure headaches is in the hand.

Amitriptyline: Antidepressant drug; brand name Elavil.

Amulet: Object, especially a charm, worn to ward off evil spirits or perform other magical functions.

Analgesic: A drug that relieves pain.

Anticoagulant: Substance that slows blood clotting.

Antidepressant: Medication that relieves depression.

Antihistamine: Substance that neutralizes the action of histamine or inhibits its production in the body.

Arachnoid membrane: The middle of three coverings on the brain.

Aspirin: Common name for acetylsalicylic acid.

Atropine: A white alkaloid substance used to treat heart and eye ailments, obtained from the plant *Atropa belladonna*.

Aura: The nervous-system disturbances that precede an attack of classical migraine.

Aura mater: The tough outer coating of the brain.

Baclofen: A drug to relieve spasticity (abnormally contracted muscles) and sometimes used to treat tic douloureux; brand name Lioresal.

Benign: Not dangerous or harmful.

Beta blocker: A drug that inhibits activity in certain nervous-system pathways.

Biofeedback: The conscious monitoring of information about usually unconscious bodily processes, such as heart rate or blood pressure; can be used to acquire the ability to exert some control over these processes, and is often used to treat headache and migraine by some practitioners.

Bradykinin: A chemical produced when tissue is damaged; the most powerful pain-producing substance known.

Cafergot: Brand name for the migraine-treatment drug ergotamine tartrate.

Calcium channel blockers: Drugs used in the treatment of migraines.

Carbamazepine: Drug used to treat tic douloureux; brand name Tegretol.

Central nervous system: That part of the nervous system consisting of the brain and spinal cord; supervises and coordinates activity of entire nervous system.

Cerebellum: That part of the brain concerned especially with body equilibrium and coordination of movement; located at the back of the brain.

Cerebral cortex: The part of the brain where thinking occurs and perception is experienced.

Cerebrum: General name for the main portion of the brain.

Cervical spine: The part of the spine that makes up the neck.

Chiropractor: Practitioner who believes illness and pain come from incorrect positioning of bones in the spine, thus impeding normal nerve function in the nervous system; as treatment, chiropractors manipulate and adjust specific body parts such as the spinal cord.

Chlordiazepoxide: Tranquilizer; brand name Librium.

Chronic: Referring to a condition that remains present and relatively unchanged for long periods of time or one that recurs frequently.

Chronic paroxysmal hemicrania: Condition in which cluster headaches occur many times a day.

Classical migraine: Migraine headache accompanied by disturbed vision, hearing, or other sensory disorders.

Cluster headache: Recurrent stabbing pain, often near the eye, occurring most commonly in men.

Cochlear nerve: The nerve by which sound impulses are sent from the ear to the brain.

Codeine: A narcotic pain reliever.

Common migraine: Severe recurring headaches not accompanied by disturbed vision or other sensory disorders.

Concussion: Head injury that may be severe enough to cause brief unconsciousness but not permanent brain injury.

Conversion headache: Headache resulting primarily from emotional disturbance.

Convulsion: Violent, uncontrollable muscular contractions sometimes due to brain damage or nervous-system disorder.

Corticosteroid: Medication given to reduce inflammation.

Countercoup injury: Damage produced on the opposite side of the head from the side where a blow was received.

Coup injury: Damage at the spot where a blow to the head was received.

Cranium: The bony case protecting the brain.

Darvon: Brand name of propoxyphene hydrochloride, a mild narcotic analgesic.

Decongestant: Medication that shrinks swollen tissues, especially in the sinus passages.

Dihydroergotamine (DHE): Form of ergot given through a vein to treat migraine headaches.

Diazepam: Muscle relaxant and tranquilizer, marketed as Valium.

Dopamine: A chemical neurotransmitter made by the adrenal gland.

Elavil: Brand name for amitriptyline, an antidepressant drug.

Electroencephalogram (EEG): Measurement of electrical activity in the brain.

Endorphins: The body's natural opiates; in addition to having pain-relieving properties, they produce a relaxed feeling of well-being in the body.

Epidemiology: The study of how diseases occur and spread.

Equilibrium: Balance.

Ergotamine: A drug derived from grain molds, useful in treating some migraine headaches.

Exercise headache: Headache brought on by exertion.

Exorcism: Ritual believed by some to drive out demons.

Gamma-aminobutyric acid (GABA): A chemical substance that is part of the body's pain-control system; reduces nerve response to pain impulses.

Genetic: Having to do with heredity (the physical traits passed from parents to their offspring).

Ginseng: A plant whose root is thought by some to have medicinal powers.

High blood pressure: A condition in which the pressure that blood exerts on vessels and other parts of the body is too high; if left untreated, high blood pressure may be crippling or fatal.

Hypothalamus: A structure at the base of the brain that acts as a relay station for nerve impulses.

Ibuprofen: An anti-inflammatory, analgesic drug; brand names include Advil and Nuprin.

Imipramine: An antidepressant marketed as Tofranil.

Incantation: A song or chant believed to have magic or healing powers.

Inderal: Brand name for propranolol, given to prevent cluster headaches.

Indocin: Brand name for indomethacin, an anti-inflammatory drug used to treat arthritis; also used to treat chronic paroxysmal hermicrania (very frequent cluster headaches).

Librium: Brand name for chlordiazepoxide, a tranquilizer.

Limbic system: Group of structures in the brain responsible for emotions.

Lioresal: Brand name for baclofen, a drug used to treat spastic (abnormally contracted) muscles; also used against tic douloureux.

Lithium carbonate: Drug used to treat some mental illnesses.

Macho headache: Slang term for cluster headache.

Malignant: Dangerous or likely to become so; especially likely to become cancerous.

Mandible: The lower jawbone.

Maxilla: The upper jawbone.

Medulla: The part of the spinal cord that extends up into the brain.

Meprobamate: Tranquilizer; brand names Miltown and Equanil.

Methysergide: Drug that blocks serotonin; used for treatment of migraine headaches; brand name Sansert.

Migraine: A kind of headache characterized by recurrent attacks of one-sided head pain, nausea, and sometimes nervous-system symptoms such as visual or hearing disturbances.

Migraine equivalent: A condition in which nervous-system symptoms of migraine, but not the migraine headache itself, strike in recurring attacks.

Monosodium glutamate (MSG): A chemical used to heighten the taste of some foods, used especially in Chinese cooking.

Morphine: A narcotic pain reliever derived from opium.

Narcotic: A habit-forming drug that produces drowsiness, dulled thinking, and insensitivity to pain.

Nausea: The sensation of being about to vomit.

Nerve: A special cell along which nervous-system impulses move.

Neurologist: Medical physician who specializes in the structure, function, and diseases of the nervous system.

Neurology: The study of the nervous system.

Neurotransmitter: Chemical released by nerve cells that sends nerve impulses from one nerve to the next.

Nitrite: Chemical used to preserve fresh appearance or color in many processed foods, especially bacon, hot dogs, cold cuts, etc.

Nociception: A nerve's perception of damage or painful stimuli.

Nociceptor: A nerve designed to perceive painful stimuli.

Norepinephrine: A neurotransmitting chemical in the body.

Occipital bones: The bones of the back of the head.

Occipital nerve: Large nerve responsible for sensation in the back of the head.

Opium: Narcotic substance derived from the poppy plant *Papaver somniferum*. Codeine, morphine, and heroin are also derivatives of the opium poppy.

Optic nerve: Nerve that carries sight information from the eye to the brain.

Papyrus: Paper made from the papyrus reed, used by ancient Egyptians to record economic transactions and history and to inscribe literature.

Parietal bones: The upper side bones of the skull.

Percodan: Brand name for a combination of synthetic codeine and aspirin.

Peripheral nervous system: The outer branches of the nervous system; i.e., the nervous system except for the brain and spinal cord.

Phenobarbital: A narcotic tranquilizer and hypnotic (sleep medicine).

Photophobia: Intolerance or extreme sensitivity to light.

Pia mater: A delicate covering on the brain.

Placebo: A drug that has no physical mode of action but may work because the patient thinks it will.

Posttraumatic amnesia: Loss of memory that occurs after a blow to the head, wherein the victim forgets what happened just before the head was struck.

Prednisone: A steroid drug used to reduce inflammation.

Prescription: A doctor's order for a drug or therapy.

Progesterone: A steroid substance produced by the female reproductive system.

Propranolol: A drug that affects blood-vessel constriction, given to treat migraines and cluster headaches; brand name Inderal.

Prostaglandins: Chemicals that are part of the body's pain production system.

Psychological: Having to do with mental and emotional processes rather than with the physical body.

Psychophysiological: Having to do with mental, emotional, and physical processes as they work together.

Psychosomatic: Arising from mental or emotional processes rather than from physical causes.

Rebound headache: One that occurs when a vessel-constricting substance such as caffeine is not taken as usual.

Referred pain: Pain that arises in one spot but is felt in another.

Relaxation therapy: Therapy to teach relaxation and so prevent tension-caused illness and/or pain.

Reticular formation: Structure at top of spinal cord that relays nerve impulses to brain.

Reye's syndrome: A serious nervous-system disorder that can occur after contracting infectious viral disease such as influenza, especially in children and young adults who take aspirin for aches and pains of flu and flulike ailments.

Rheumatoid arthritis: A painful, inflammatory disease of the joints.

Sansert: Brand name of methysergide, a serotonin blocker used in treating migraine headaches.

Scotoma: The blind spot in the visual field that follows visual disturbances of migraine.

Secondary headache: One caused by illness or injury.

Seizure: Violent, uncontrollable muscular contraction sometimes due to brain damage or nervous-system disorder.

Serotonin: A chemical that is part of the body's pain control system; it helps regulate transmission of pain impulses.

Sinus: Hollow space inside face bones, especially near the nose.

Sinus headache: One caused when sinuses become blocked or infected and thus do not drain normally.

Skull: Bony structure of the head.

Spinal cord: Tube-shaped structure made of nervous tissue, running inside the spine; carries nerve impulses between brain and body.

Stress: Emotional pressure due to difficulties of life; also the body's reaction to such pressure.

Stroke: Sudden blockage or rupture of a blood vessel in the brain.

Subluxation: Incorrect or abnormal position, especially of vertebra.

Substance P: Chemical released in spinal cord and at tissue injury site; it activates pain nerves.

Sumatriptan: Drug used in the treatment of migraines and cluster headaches; brand name Imitrex.

Tegretol: Brand name for carbamazepine, drug for treatment of tic douloureux.

Temperomandibular joint: Hinged joint linking jawbone to head.

TENS: Transcutaneous electrical nerve stimulation, a technique for blocking pain impulses with tiny electrical shocks.

Tension headache: One arising from various causes, including anxiety and chronic muscle constriction.

Thalamus: Structure in brain that recognizes nerve impulses as pain.

Tic douloureux: Chronic, painful spasm of the face, arising from irritation of trigeminal nerve.

Tranquilizer: Medication that decreases anxiety.

Trephination: Technique of opening the skull, done in ancient times to release evil spirits; now done to relieve pressure on brain.

Trigeminal nerve: One of the head's main nerves, responsible for sensation and pain impulses in the face, scalp, and skull.

Tumor: A growth of abnormal tissue.

Tympanic membrane: The eardrum.

Tyramine: A chemical present in chocolate, cheese, and some other foods; may cause migraine headaches.

Valium: Brand name for diazepam, a muscle relaxant and tranquilizer.

Vascular headache: One arising from swollen or otherwise abnormal blood vessels in the head.

Vertebra: One of the bones of the spine.

Vertigo: Dizziness.

Visual cortex: The structure in the brain that receives and interprets nerve impulses from the eyes.

APPENDIX

INDEX

APPENDIX

PICTURE CREDITS

Mary Kittredge, a former associate editor of the medical journal *Respiratory Care,* is a freelance writer of nonfiction and fiction. She is certified as a respiratory-care technician by the American Association for Respiratory Therapy. She has been a member of the respiratory-care staff at Yale-New Haven Hospital and Medical Center since 1972. Ms. Kittredge was educated at Trinity College, Hartford, and the University of California Medical Center, San Francisco. She is the author of *The Respiratory System* in the Chelsea House 21ST CENTURY HEALTH AND WELLNESS series, and of young-adult biographies *Marc Antony, Frederick the Great,* and *Jane Addams.* Her writing awards include the Ruell Crompton Tuttle Essay Prize and the Mystery Writers of America Robert L. Fish Award for best first short-mystery fiction.

Sandra L. Thurman, a graduate of Mercer University, is the Director of the Office of National AIDS Policy at the White House. For more than a decade, Ms. Thurman has been a leader and advocate for people with AIDS at the local, state, and federal levels. From 1988 to 1993, Ms. Thurman served as the Executive Director of AID Atlanta, a community-based nonprofit organization that provides health and support services to people living with HIV/AIDS. From 1993 to 1996, Ms. Thurman was the Director of Advocacy Programs at the Task Force for Child Survival and Development at the Carter Center in Atlanta, Georgia. Most recently, she served as the Director of Citizen Exchanges at the United States Information Agency. She is a recognized expert on AIDS issues and has provided testimony before the United States Senate, the White House Conference on HIV/AIDS, and the National Commission on AIDS.

C. Everett Koop, M.D., Sc.D., currently serves as chairman of the board of his own website, www.drkoop.com, and is the Elizabeth DeCamp McInerny professor at Dartmouth College, from which he graduated in 1937. Dr. Koop received his doctor of medicine degree from Cornell Medical College in 1941 and his doctor of science degree from the University of Pennsylvania in 1947. A pediatric surgeon of international reputation, he was previously surgeon in chief of Children's Hospital of Philadelphia and professor of pediatric surgery and pediatrics at the University of Pennsylvania. A former U.S. Surgeon General, Dr. Koop was also the director of the Office of International Health. He has served as surgery editor of the *Journal of Clinical Pediatrics* and editor in chief of the *Journal of Pediatric Surgery.* In his more than 60 years of experience in health care, government, and industry, Dr. Koop has received numerous awards and honors, including 35 honorary degrees.